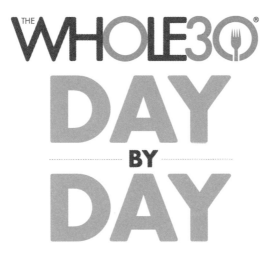

THE WHOLE30®

DAY

BY

DAY

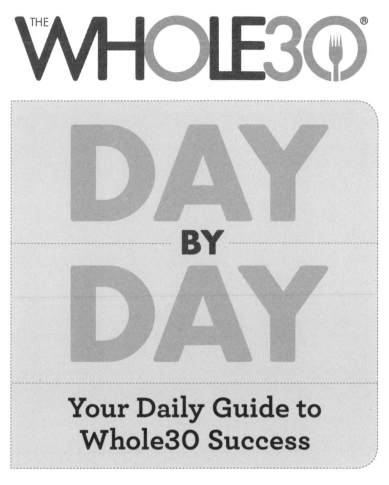

THE WHOLE30®

DAY BY DAY

Your Daily Guide to
Whole30 Success

MELISSA HARTWIG

Houghton Mifflin Harcourt
BOSTON NEW YORK 2017

For my son. Tonight, I am thankful for you.

For information about permission to reproduce selections from this book,
write to trade.permissions@hmhco.com or to Permissions,
Houghton Mifflin Harcourt Publishing Company,
3 Park Avenue, 19th floor, New York, New York 10016.

hmhco.com

Library of Congress Cataloging-in-Publication Data is available.

ISBN 978-1-328-83923-7 (paperback)

ISBN 978-1-328-83930-5 (ebook)

Cover and interior design by Vertigo Design NYC

Illustrations by Virginia de Vries

Printed in China

SCP 10 9 8 7 6 5 4 3 2 1

CONTENTS

ACKNOWLEDGMENTS

To Justin Schwartz, my editor at Houghton Mifflin Harcourt, your support in this project has been especially meaningful. Thank you for getting as excited about these pages as I was, and then helping me make them even better.

To Bruce Nichols, Ellen Archer, Marina Padakis, Claire Safran, Jessica Gilo, Adriana Rizzo, and the entire Houghton Mifflin Harcourt team, on behalf of my Whole30 community, thank you. You have helped me change so many lives, and I am forever grateful.

To Andrea Magyar and Trish Bunnett at Penguin Canada, thank you for your continued support of the Whole30 program. Our Canadian community is lucky to have you on our team.

To Christy Fletcher, it's incredible to look at what we've done together. Thank you for always being in my corner, and caring so much about our mission and the people we serve.

To Grainne Fox, Melissa Chinchillo, Erin McFadden, Sylvie Greenberg, Sarah Fuentes, and the Fletcher and Company team, thank you for lending your expertise to these books and my engagements.

To my Whole30 team: Kristen Crandall, Shanna Keller, Jen Kendall, Karyn Scott, and Tawni Schall; thank you for your help and encouragement on this book, and for holding down the whole darn fort while I wrote it. You are the heart and soul of Whole30.

To Virginia de Vries, thank you for bringing this book to life with your creativity and talent. It looks more beautiful than I ever could have imagined, and that is all thanks to you. I am so grateful to have you on our team.

To my April 2017 Whole30 Facebook group—YOU are here in these pages. Your hard work, dedication, grace, and generosity in sharing your experience, it's all been captured here. Without you, this book would not have been possible. Thank you for giving so much of yourselves to this community, and this project.

To my family and friends, you are my biggest cheerleaders, and I am grateful to have you to lean on. To my mom, who has surely bought a dozen copies of everything I've ever written, I love you.

To my son, you are my whole world. All of this is for you. I love you inside-out.

Finally, to YOU, my Whole30ers . . . you give so much more to me than I could ever give to you. You have all my love and support, heart emoji.

PREFACE

SINCE THE PROGRAM'S CREATION IN 2009, I've written or co-authored six books about the Whole30, all of which I consider my book-babies. The process of bringing each one to life was meaningful and rewarding in its own way; true labors of love, equal parts frustrating and exhilarating. As a parent, I know I'm not supposed to have favorites . . . but if you promise not to tell the other books, this one holds a special place in my heart. I've had the idea for *The Whole30 Day by Day* for years, but this was not the kind of book I could just sit down and write. If I was going to guide you through the Whole30 one day at a time, making sure my recommendations, tips, and strategies were timely and effective for as many of you as possible, I needed to do my research.

So I did. For more than three years, I studied you and your Whole30 journey. Which days are the hardest, where do you need a swift dose of tough love, how many times should I remind you to eat more? At what point, specifically, do you transition from "Why is this so hard?" to "I could do this forever!"? Which parts scare you the most, when could you use a good laugh, and how many days does Kill All the Things *really* last?

I followed you on social media, comparing your experience to our original Whole30 Timeline. I casually posed questions: "Are you dreaming about food yet?" We posted short surveys: "Did you eat All the Things on Day 31, or did you feel too good to throw yourself down the junk food aisle?" I searched your hashtags, wondering when and under what circumstances #whole30fail was most likely to show up.

My research culminated in April 2017, when I led hundreds of people through a group Whole30 on my Facebook page. I connected with them twice a day for 30 days, asking what they needed to stay motivated, inspired, and accountable; posing advice I thought would be helpful; and logging their responses.

Only then did I begin to write, starting with Day 1: Welcome to the Whole30. Let me give you a pep talk. Here is what you need to focus on today. Look to these resources for help. Take these steps to make tomorrow as successful as possible. When I went back and read what I had written, I got goosebumps. More than three years of research, distilled down to just six pages—six pages that will play a huge part in your Whole30 success story.

How could this book *not* be my favorite?

I hope you love the process of working through *The Whole30 Day by Day* as much as I enjoyed the process of creating it for you. Welcome to the Whole30; I'm so happy you're here.

Best in health,
Melissa

HOW TO USE THIS BOOK

I THINK OF THIS BOOK as the companion guide to *The Whole30*; the icing on that book's "how to" cake. Which is actually a really bad analogy given the rules of the Whole30, but "the mashed potatoes on the meatloaf" doesn't translate as nicely. *The Whole30* is all about the practical application of the program: "eat this, not that," and "plan like this, prep like that." It gives you a taste of what to expect during your 30 days but doesn't dive deep into the daily challenges, emotional ups and downs, and physical variables you're likely to experience on the program.

This companion guide is very, very different. I've observed hundreds of thousands of people do the Whole30 since 2009, and everything I know about the program, the people who complete it, and the results they achieve went in this book. Consider it your field manual for the Whole30, helping you plan and prepare; guiding you through the program with motivation, support, and resources specific to each day; and taking you straight through the mission-critical reintroduction period.

I'll start you off on Day 0, with basic planning and preparation guidance and action items to set yourself up for Whole30 success. Then, when you're ready, you'll turn the page to Day 1, diving into the heart of *The Whole30 Day by Day*—a comprehensive guide to every day of your Whole30 journey.

Each day is broken down into seven sections, designed to be read as part of your morning routine.

- **TIMELINE:** This section explains what you might expect to feel and experience during that day; physically, mentally, and emotionally. While every day may not exactly match your experience, our timeline has proven to be a tongue-in-cheek but eerily accurate predictor of a typical Whole30 journey. During your first Whole30 (especially the first ten days), it really does help knowing that what you are going through is normal and expected, even if you are a little bit ahead of or behind the curve.

→ **MELISSA'S MOTIVATION:** Imagine every morning when you wake up, I'm sitting at the foot of your bed, giving you the Whole30 pep talk you need to get up and conquer your day. Okay—while that may sound more creepy than motivating, this is where I talk directly to you, giving you encouragement, support, and tough love where needed. If this section makes you tearful, prompts a fist-pump, or makes you mad at me (because you don't like it, but you know I'm right), I've done my job here.

→ **FAQ:** Here's where I'll answer a commonly asked question relevant to this phase of your Whole30. While I'll keep my responses pretty high-level, know that each question posed here has a more detailed answer in *The Whole30*. If you need more information after reading, crack it open, but if you've thoroughly read *The Whole30*, these timely reminders should be all that is needed to help you stay on track.

→ **COMMUNITY INSPIRATION:** I've hand-picked some of my favorite quotes from Whole30ers throughout all stages of the program to inspire you every day. They're funny, relatable, and most of all, designed to remind you that you are not alone in this life-changing experience—past and present Whole30ers have been and will be right there with you, just as I am.

➤ **TIP:** In this section, I'll give you practical tips for navigating each phase of your Whole30. This is nitty-gritty stuff—things to do, pay attention to, and plan for—keeping you on track, well-fed, motivated, and confident in your new lifestyle. These tips will come in handy well beyond that specific day, so flag your favorites and return to them often.

➤ **HACK:** My favorite section to research, these "hacks" all come straight from habit and willpower science. They're designed to help you take advantage of the way your brain works, easing you around trouble spots; giving you the tools you need to cement your new, healthy habits; and preparing you for potential life-after-Whole30 pitfalls.

➤ **EXTRA CREDIT:** "Homework" sounds like drudgery, so I decided to appeal to your inner overachiever and call it "extra credit." These recommendations are all carefully designed to help you plan for the following day. While all of the guided self-reflections in this handbook are optional, you really should spend some time on this section. If there was one thing you could do to reduce stress, increase your self-confidence, and maximize your Whole30 results, it's these extra credit assignments.

There are also three pages of guided self-reflection for every day of the program, designed to be completed as part of your evening routine, while the events and your feelings about them are still fresh in your mind. I've gently encouraged you to focus on a particular area of your Whole30 practice each day, and I've used habit research to design this section, too. Completing these pages will help you stay on track, maintain your commitment, and increase your motivation for the following day—plus they'll help you clearly see your progress day-to-day, from one week to the next, and looking back at the end of your program. You can even refer to these entries during your *next* Whole30, which will help you clearly see the dramatic nature of the lifestyle changes you've made and maintained between programs.

As part of your nightly reflections, you'll also track your non-scale victories (NSVs)—energy, sleep, cravings, and anything else you checked off as important to you when preparing for the program. In the text, I often encourage you to be generous here; progress is progress, and on the Whole30, small improvements add up to huge, life-changing results come Day 30. This section also serves to remind you that you're here to change your *health, habits, and relationship with food*—so don't even worry about the scale, because that's not what's important.

There's also space to log your Whole30 meals, so when food boredom sets in, you can easily keep things fresh by pulling out an old favorite. Being thorough here will also come in handy if you experience digestive symptoms, cravings, or other unfavorable effects along the way, serving as a food journal to help you pinpoint the culprit and make adjustments to tomorrow's plan.

Finally, there's a box you'll need to check at the end of every successful Whole30 day, celebrating being one step closer to your food freedom and strengthening your commitment. I can't actually *see* when you check the box, but knowing someone (or in this case, something) expects you to follow through is often enough to get you past a tough point. So on that note, I expect those boxes *will* be checked—even if that's the only thing you do before crawling into bed at 8 p.m. on the evening of Day 3.

And then . . . hooray! You're a Whole30 alumnus, looking and feeling better than you have in years (decades? EVER?) and ready to start living your food freedom. But first, *you must reintroduce*. Reintroduction—the part where you systematically add foods back in and compare your experiences—is half of the Whole30 learning experience and can't be skipped or cut short. But reintroduction can also be kind of confusing to figure out on your own, and after 30 days of strict rules, having a little guidance as you bring foods back in can be comforting—so I'm going to walk you through this part, too.

At the end of *The Whole30 Day by Day*, you'll find a separate section with Fast Track and Slow Roll reintroduction guidelines, sample schedules, and space for you to record your reintroduction food choices and the results of your experiment. There is also extra room to journal an extended reintro period—the slower you take this phase, the more you'll learn, and the better prepared you'll be to make the right choices for you in your food freedom. Use our templates or create your own, finishing the program strong and closing the book out with one final high-five from me to you.

Back in 2009, when I was writing the very first blog post about my 30-day dietary self-experiment, I called the program "Change Your Life in 30 Days." While it didn't exactly roll off the tongue, the title has more than proven itself accurate over the years—and I'm excited for you to prove this true for yourself. Whether this is your first Whole30 or your seventh, I hope you use *The Whole30 Day by Day* to change your own life. Keep it close by. Mark it up with pens, highlighters, and markers. Add bookmarks and tabs to your favorite pages. Dog-ear them, if that's your thing. (I do it too; it makes my books feel well-loved.) And don't be embarrassed if at some point you notice a ghee or mayo stain on the cover, because that's officially how *all* Whole30ers christen their books.

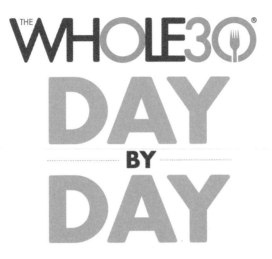

PROGRAM RULES

✓ Yes. Eat real food.

Eat moderate portions of meat, seafood, and eggs; lots of vegetables; some fruit; plenty of natural fats; and herbs, spices, and seasonings. Eat foods with very few ingredients, all pronounceable ingredients or, better yet, no ingredients listed at all because they're whole and unprocessed.

✗ No. For 30 days:

➡ DO NOT CONSUME ADDED SUGAR, REAL OR ARTIFICIAL. No maple syrup, honey, agave nectar, coconut sugar, date syrup, stevia, Splenda, Equal, Nutrasweet, xylitol, etc. Read your labels, because companies sneak sugar into products in ways you might not recognize.

➡ DO NOT CONSUME ALCOHOL IN ANY FORM, NOT EVEN IN COOKING. (And ideally, no tobacco products of any sort, either.)

➡ DO NOT EAT GRAINS. This includes (but is not limited to) wheat, rye, barley, oats, corn, rice, millet, bulgur, sorghum, sprouted grains, and all gluten-free pseudo-cereals like quinoa, amaranth, and buckwheat. This also includes all the ways we add wheat, corn, and rice into our foods in the form of bran, germ, starch, and so on. Again, read your labels.

➡ DO NOT EAT LEGUMES. This includes beans of all kinds (black, red, pinto, navy, white, kidney, lima, fava, etc.), peas, chickpeas, lentils, and peanuts. No peanut butter, either. This also includes all forms of soy—soy sauce, miso, tofu, tempeh, edamame, and all the ways they sneak soy into foods (like lecithin).

➡️ **DO NOT EAT DAIRY.** This includes cow, goat, or sheep's milk products like milk, cream, cheese, kefir, yogurt, sour cream, ice cream, or frozen yogurt.

➡️ **DO NOT CONSUME CARRAGEENAN, MSG, OR SULFITES.** If these ingredients appear in any form on the label of your processed food or beverage, it's out for the Whole30.

➡️ **DO NOT CONSUME BAKED GOODS, JUNK FOODS, OR TREATS WITH "APPROVED" INGREDIENTS.** Recreating or buying sweets, treats, and foods-with-no-brakes (even if the ingredients are technically compliant) is totally missing the point of the Whole30, and will compromise your life-changing results. These are the same foods that got you into health trouble in the first place—and a pancake is still a pancake, even if it's made with coconut flour.

* *Some specific foods that fall under this rule include: pancakes, waffles, bread, tortillas, biscuits, muffins, cupcakes, cookies, brownies, pizza crust, cereal, and ice cream. No commercially-prepared chips (potato, tortilla, plantain, etc.) or French fries either. However, this list is not limited strictly to these items— there may be other foods that you find are not psychologically healthy for your Whole30. Use your best judgment with those foods that aren't on this list, but that you suspect are not helping you change your habits or break those cravings. Our mantra: When in doubt, leave it out. It's only 30 days.*

ONE LAST AND FINAL RULE: Do not step on the scale or take any body measurements for 30 days. The Whole30 is about so much more than weight loss, and to focus only on body composition means you'll overlook all of the other dramatic, lifelong benefits this plan has to offer. So, no weighing yourself, analyzing body fat, or taking comparative measurements during your Whole30. (We do encourage you to weigh yourself before and after, so you can see one of the more tangible results of your efforts when your program is over.)

the fine print . . .

*These foods are exceptions to the rule and
are allowed during your Whole30.*

✓ GHEE OR CLARIFIED BUTTER

These are the only sources of dairy allowed during your Whole30.
Plain old butter is NOT allowed, as the milk proteins found in
non-clarified butter could impact the results of your program.

✓ FRUIT JUICE

Some products or recipes will include fruit juice as a stand-alone
ingredient or natural sweetener, which is fine for the purposes of
the Whole30. (We have to draw the line somewhere.)

✓ CERTAIN LEGUMES

Green beans, sugar snap peas, and snow peas are allowed.
While they're technically legumes, these are far more "pod" than
"bean," and green plant matter is generally good for you.

✓ VINEGAR

Nearly all forms of vinegar, including white, red wine, balsamic, apple cider, and rice, are allowed during your Whole30 program. (The only exception is malt vinegar, which generally
contains gluten.)

✓ COCONUT AMINOS

All brands of coconut aminos (a brewed and naturally fermented
soy sauce substitute) are acceptable, even if you see the word
"coconut nectar" in the ingredient list.

✓ SALT

Did you know that all iodized table salt contains sugar? Sugar
(often in the form of dextrose) is chemically essential to keep
the potassium iodide from oxidizing and being lost. Because all
restaurants and pre-packaged foods contain salt, we're making
salt an exception to our "no added sugar" rule.

4

TOUGH LOVE

This is for those of you who are considering taking on this life-changing month, but aren't sure you can actually pull it off, cheat-free, for a full 30 days. This is for the people who have tried this before, but who "slipped" or "fell off the wagon" or "just HAD to eat (fill in food) because of this (fill in event)." This is for you.

This is not hard. Don't you dare tell us this is hard. Beating cancer is hard. Birthing a baby is hard. Losing a parent is hard. Drinking your coffee black. Is. Not. Hard. You've done harder things than this, and you have no excuse not to complete the program as written. It's only thirty days, and it's for the most important health cause on earth—the only physical body you will have in this lifetime.

Don't even consider the possibility of a "slip." Unless you physically trip and your face lands in a pizza, there is no "slip." It is always a choice to eat something off-plan. Commit to the program 100% for the full 30 days. Don't give yourself an excuse to fail before you've even begun.

You never, ever have to eat anything you don't want to eat. You're all big boys and girls. Toughen up. Say, "No, thank you." Stick to your guns. Just because it's your sister's birthday or your best friend's wedding or your company picnic does not mean you *have* to eat anything. It is always a choice, and we would hope you stopped succumbing to peer pressure in 7th grade.

This does require effort. Grocery shopping, meal planning, dining out, social situations, and cravings will all prove challenging at some point during your program. We've given you tools, advice, and resources to succeed, but you must take responsibility for your own Whole30. Improved health, fitness, and quality of life doesn't happen automatically just because you're taking a pass on bread.

YOU CAN DO THIS. You've come too far to back out now. You want to do this. You need to do this. And we know that you are READY to do this.

MEAL TEMPLATE

Practice good mealtime habits. Eat meals at the table in a relaxed fashion. Do not allow distractions like TV, phone, or email while you are eating. Chew slowly and thoroughly—don't gulp. Take the time to enjoy the delicious, healthy food you have prepared!

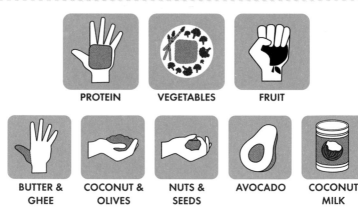

PROTEIN	VEGETABLES	FRUIT		
BUTTER & GHEE	COCONUT & OLIVES	NUTS & SEEDS	AVOCADO	COCONUT MILK

Eat three meals a day, starting with a good breakfast. Base each meal around 1–2 palm-sized protein sources. Fill the rest of your plate with vegetables. Occasionally add a serving of fruit. Add fat in the following recommended amounts per meal:

All oils and cooking fats (olive oil, animal fats, etc.):
1–2 thumb-sized portions

All butters (ghee, coconut butter, nut butters, etc.):
1–2 thumb-sized portions

Coconut (shredded or flaked):
1–2 open (heaping) handfuls

Olives:
1–2 open (heaping) handfuls

Nuts and seeds:
Up to one closed handful

Avocado: ½–1 (whole) avocado

Coconut milk: Between ¼ and ½ of one (14-oz.) can

Make each meal large enough to satisfy you until the next meal—snack only when necessary. Stop eating a few hours before bed.

⫶I—I⫶ FUELING FOR EXERCISE

Eat 15–75 minutes pre-workout, as a signal to prepare your body for activity. If you train first thing in the morning, something is better than nothing. Choose foods that are easily digestible and palatable. This is the most variable factor in our template, so experiment with different foods, quantities, and timing.

pre-workout

✓ Include a small amount of protein (½ a meal size or smaller)

✓ (optionally) a small amount of fat (½ a meal size or smaller)

✗ Do not add fruit or carb-dense vegetables to your pre-workout snack.

Eat *immediately* following exercise (15–30 minutes).

post-workout

✓ Eat a meal-sized easily digestible protein.

✓ The appropriate amount of carb-dense vegetables (based on the Carb Curve in *It Starts With Food*, page 244).

✗ Do not use fruit as your primary post-workout carb.

✗ Add little to no fat.

Examples of carb-dense vegetables appropriate for post-workout include sweet potatoes/yams, taro/poi, butternut squash, acorn squash, pumpkin, or beets.

> Note, your PWO meal is a special bonus meal—not meant to replace breakfast, lunch, or dinner. Think of it as a necessary source of additional nutrients, designed to help you recover faster and more efficiently from high-intensity exercise.

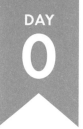

DAY 0

WELCOME TO THE WHOLE30! Today (or however long you need to get ready) is all about planning and preparation. We know you're excited and want to jump right in while motivation is high, but habit research shows that those who move from thinking about a change straight into action (skipping preparation) are more likely to abandon their efforts when the going gets tough. Full disclosure: The Whole30 CAN get tough.

So channel that motivation into your planning and prep, because there really is no such thing as *too prepared* on the Whole30. We'll give you extra reflection and planning space today to help you choose a start date, get your house in order, and more before your all-important Day 1.

Melissa's Motivation

I'm so happy you've joined us! Whether you're looking to improve symptoms, have more energy, sleep better, relieve digestive distress, or conquer your cravings, you're in the right place.

You've noticed the Whole30 looks different from anything you've done before. The Whole30 is way more than a "diet"; resetting your health from the inside out and prompting you to create new habits and restore a healthy emotional relationship with food. Over the next 30 days, you'll find yourself challenged physically and mentally. But if you work the program and stay connected to your support team and our community, the next 30 days have the potential to deliver radical and permanent change. You will discover how amazing your body can feel. Your confidence will spill over in every area of your life. And at the end, you will know true food freedom. The Whole30 is *that* powerful—and if you've made it this far, YOU ARE READY for this change.

In a 2016 survey of 8,000 Whole30 graduates, 88% said the Whole30 really did change their lives!

PLAN & PREPARE

0

For detailed guidance, see pages 17–31 in *The Whole30*.

CHOOSE YOUR START DATE Find a 30-day period when you don't have something mega-important going on, like your own wedding or a once-in-a-lifetime vacation. A birthday party or routine business trip is NOT reason to put it off! Then add 10 days at the end for reintroduction.

Write your start date down here: ....

ACTION ITEM: *Go public! Accountability is important to Whole30 success, so post your start date on Facebook, share it on your blog, email your friends, and tell your family.*

BUILD YOUR SUPPORT TEAM You'll need help to see this commitment through—people to motivate you, answer your questions, and be a cheerleader when the going gets tough. If you're doing the Whole30 with a buddy or as part of a group, great! If not, find family members, friends, or co-workers to be your accountability, recipe resource, or Whole30 mentor.

ACTION ITEM: *Connect with the Whole30 community and team on social media and the free Whole30 Forum (forum. whole30.com), where you'll find Whole30ers willing to listen, help, and offer advice day and night.*

GET YOUR HOUSE READY First, clean all the junk out of your pantry. (Yes, you really need to do this.) Then, plan your first week of meals, just-in-case snacks, and emergency food. Finally, go grocery shopping and stock up on essentials (like ghee and coconut milk) and what you'll need for your first few meals.

ACTION ITEM: *Sign up for Real Plans (w30.co/w30realplans) to create a fully customizable Whole30 meal plan, automatic shopping list, and generated meal prep instructions in 15 minutes.*

9

PLAN & PREPARE ◀━━━

━━➤ **IF/THEN PLANS** Think ahead to potentially stressful or challenging situations (like a business lunch or family road trip) and create an if/then plan for handling each one. The "if/then" structure is based on habit research, helping you recognize scenarios that could trip you up in the moment and manage them more effectively.

ACTION ITEM: *IF people ask what this "new diet" is all about, THEN you'll say . . . ? Use our ideas on page 13 to get you started, then rework it in your own words (or just steal ours—we don't mind).*

━━➤ **TOSS THE SCALE** Since you can't weigh yourself during the Whole30, you need to remove the temptation. Stick it in the garage, give it to a friend to "hold," or donate it to charity— just get it out of the bathroom.

ACTION ITEM: *Look at our LONG list of non-scale victories (NSVs) starting on page 16, and highlight or circle the ones that are the most important to you. These are WAY more important for your health and happiness than the measurement of your gravitational pull!*

━━➤ **TAKE STARTING STATS** Take Day 0 calibrations, like your body weight, body fat %, measurements (bust, waist, hips, etc.), and photos. Wear the same clothes and stand in the same spot in all photos, shooting from the front, back, and side, including a close-up of your face. You can also take photos of things like your skin or joint swelling for comparison.

ACTION ITEM: *Record your Day 0 statistics here:*

WHOLE30 PLANNING & PREPARATION

Use this space to recruit your Whole30 support team, making note of who you'll ask for help and what role they will play for you. (See our examples for inspiration.)

MOM: Cheerleader! Sends me texts every day asking how it's going and saying, "Good job!"

BEST FRIEND: Tough love. On-call in case I feel like bailing or need to vent.

CO-WORKER: Recipe resource. She's got a ton of Whole30 experience, I'll ask for help if I get bored.

CREATE YOUR DAY 1 WHOLE30 MEAL PLAN AND
A SHOPPING LIST OF THE BASICS YOU'LL NEED TO
GET YOUR KITCHEN WHOLE30-FRIENDLY.
(Skip this if you're using Real Plans—they'll do it all for you.)

CREATE YOUR IF/THEN PLANS, USING OUR PROMPTS
TO GET YOU STARTED.

IF I'm stuck late at work/in traffic/at the game, THEN I'll ...

....

....

....

....

....

....

....

IF I'm at happy hour and offered a drink, THEN I'll ...

....

....

....

....

....

....

....

IF there's nothing compliant to eat at the party, THEN I'll ...

....

....

....

....

....

....

....

IF my friends tease me about my "crazy diet," THEN I'll ...

_____

_____

_____

_____

_____

_____

_____

_____

_____

_____

Create your own if/then plans here:

_____

_____

_____

_____

_____

_____

_____

_____

_____

_____

_____

_____

_____

_____

WHAT IS THE WHOLE30?

You'll hear this question often; how will you answer it? Here are a few options, but add your own take on the Whole30 here. Note: You'll expand your "elevator pitch" even more on Day 9.

"The Whole30 is a 30-day experiment designed to help me figure out how the foods I'm eating are affecting me. I pull commonly problematic foods out for 30 days, then reintroduce them one at a time and compare my experience."

"They call the Whole30 a 'reset,' not a diet. It's not about weight loss; there's no calorie counting or restriction. I'm using it to learn how food affects me, create new habits, and lose my sugar cravings."

"The Whole30 is a 30 day program designed to improve my cravings, metabolism, digestion, and overall health. I'm trying it to improve my energy, sleep better, and ditch my nighttime ice cream habit."

NON-SCALE VICTORIES

Here is a very, very long list of the Whole30 benefits you may have experienced. (And we're sure you'll find a few that aren't detailed here!) We call these "non-scale victories"—in fact, that phrase even has its own hashtag (#NSV) on social media because we believe it's so critical to evaluating your Whole30 results. So take a moment (before you get on that scale) to check off everything you've noticed in the last 30 days. Be generous here—you worked hard, and you deserve to be proud of what you've accomplished!

Mood, Emotion, and Psychology

- Happier
- More outgoing
- More patient
- More optimistic
- Laugh more
- Less anxious
- Less stressed
- Handling stress better
- Your kids say you're more fun
- Fewer mood swings
- Improved behavior (kids)
- Fewer tantrums (kids)
- Less depression
- Improved mental health
- Fewer sugar cravings
- Fewer carb cravings
- Improved body image
- Improved self-esteem
- Improved self-confidence
- Less reliance on the scale
- Feeling in control of your food

Physical (Outside)

- Fewer blemishes
- Glowing skin
- No more under-eye circles
- Improvement in rashes or patches
- Less dimpled skin
- Longer, stronger nails
- Stronger, thicker hair
- Brighter eyes
- Fresher breath
- Whiter teeth
- Flatter stomach
- Leaner appearance
- Clothes fitting better
- Wedding ring fitting better
- Less bloating
- More defined muscle tone
- Less joint swelling
- Looking younger
- Feeling more confident in your appearance

Physical (Inside)

- Healthier gums
- Less stiff joints
- Less painful joints
- Fewer PMS symptoms
- A more regular monthly cycle
- Increased libido
- Less stomach pain
- Less diarrhea
- Less constipation
- Less gas
- Less bloating
- Improved "regularity"
- Not getting sick as often
- Fewer seasonal allergies
- Reduction in food allergies
- Fewer migraines
- Fewer asthma attacks
- Less acid reflux
- Less heartburn
- Less chronic pain
- Less chronic fatigue
- Less tendonitis/bursitis
- Less shoulder/back/knee pain
- Improved blood pressure
- Improved cholesterol numbers
- Improved circulation
- Improved blood sugar regulation
- Improved medical symptoms
- Reduced or eliminated medications
- Recovering faster from injury or illness

Food and Behaviors

- Healthier relationship with food
- Improved disordered eating habits
- No more binging
- Practicing mindful eating
- Learned how to read a label
- Eats to satiety
- Listens to your body
- Abandoned yo-yo or crash dieting
- No longer afraid of dietary fat
- Learned how to cook
- No longer use food for comfort
- No longer use food as reward
- No longer use food as punishment
- No longer use food as love
- No longer a slave to sugar/carbs
- Can identify cravings vs. hunger
- Fewer cravings
- Healthy strategies to deal with cravings
- More nutrition in your diet
- Food no longer has unwanted "side effects"
- No more food guilt or shame

Brain Function

- [ ] Improved attention span
- [ ] Improved performance at job or school
- [ ] Improved memory
- [ ] Faster reaction times
- [ ] Fewer ADD/ADHD symptoms
- [ ] Thinking more clearly
- [ ] Feeling generally more productive

Sleep

- [ ] Sleeping more
- [ ] Falling asleep more easily
- [ ] Sleeping more soundly
- [ ] No longer need a sleep aid
- [ ] No more "snooze" button
- [ ] Awakening feeling refreshed
- [ ] Less snoring
- [ ] Less night sweats
- [ ] Less sleep apnea
- [ ] Fewer night cramps

Energy

- [ ] Energy levels are higher
- [ ] Energy levels are more even
- [ ] More energy in the morning
- [ ] No more mid-day energy slump
- [ ] More energy to play with your kids
- [ ] More energy to exercise
- [ ] More energy to socialize
- [ ] More energy at work or school
- [ ] No longer need to eat every two hours
- [ ] No longer get cranky if you don't eat
- [ ] Feel energetic between meals
- [ ] Need less sugar or caffeine

Sport, Exercise, and Play

- [ ] Started moving or exercising
- [ ] Became more consistent with exercise
- [ ] Can exercise longer, harder, or faster
- [ ] Feel more athletic
- [ ] Can lift heavier things
- [ ] Hit new "personal bests"
- [ ] Recover more effectively
- [ ] Trying new activities
- [ ] Play more with your kids or dog
- [ ] More coordinated
- [ ] Balance is better
- [ ] Outside more

Lifestyle and Social

- New healthy habits to teach your kids
- More knowledgeable about nutrition
- Shop locally and eat seasonally
- New cooking skills
- New recipes
- Meal prep is organized and efficient
- Made new like-minded friends who support your lifestyle
- Maximize your food budget
- Spend less time and money at the doctor's office
- Created other health goals
- Healthy eating habits have brought your family closer
- Joined a new community
- Your kids have the best school lunches
- People ask you what you're doing differently
- People come to you for health, food, or lifestyle advice

 I am Whole30.

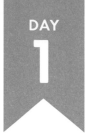

DAY 1

WELCOME TO DAY 1 of your Whole30. You're really doing it (changing your life), and it's all *so very exciting!* You added nutpods to your morning coffee and confidently skipped the sugar while you happily ate a slice of frittata. You packed a protein salad for lunch (plus some emergency food just in case), and there's a beef and sweet potato chili simmering in your slow cooker at home. This Whole30 stuff is a breeze!

Then, out of nowhere, you're hit with a crippling panic. What have I done? Can I really do this for 30 days? Who is going to do all these dishes? You're overwhelmed. You're anxious. You're *hungry.* All of a sudden, you're not so sure this was a good idea.

RELAX. Of course this is a good idea! It's normal to have mixed feelings on the first day. Share your excitement when you're excited, but allow yourself to feel nervous, too. Just remember you have a great plan, lots of support, and some fantastic resources to see you through.

Melissa's Motivation

Today you need a pep talk—something to inspire you and remind you why you started. So here you go: You are EXACTLY where you need to be. Here on this page; Day 1 of your Whole30 journey. Whatever it took to get here; however many times you've stumbled before; no matter how much self-doubt, anxiety, or skepticism you hold, you are HERE NOW for a reason.

Because you remembered that you are worth it. Because you need a big win in your life. Because you may not get another chance. Because you are ready to regain control. Because you believe that honoring this commitment to your own health and happiness will change *everything.* Because you *deserve* the kind of food freedom the Whole30 can bring.

Today is your DAY ONE, not just for the Whole30, but for the rest of your life. And we will do this together, one day at a time.

FAQ

WHERE CAN I FIND MEAL PLANNING HELP? Meal planning is a necessity on the Whole30. You'll stress less, spend less time in the grocery store, and save money buying only the foods you need for the week. There are three routes to Whole30 meal planning:

➤ **REAL PLANS (w30.co/w30realplans):** This online Whole30 meal-planning service with more than 1,000 compliant recipes will help you plan 30 days of meals in under 10 minutes, and generate automatic shopping lists and meal prep instructions. Plus it's fully customizable, so you'll only plan for the meals you want, and can eliminate any ingredients to which you are allergic or just don't like. Our Whole30ers overwhelmingly love this service, and they're using it well after their Whole30 is over to save time and money.

➤ **THE 7-DAY MEAL PLAN IN *THE WHOLE30*:** We give you a one-week meal plan with day-by-day meal prep instructions starting on page 196, using the simple recipes found in the book. After a week of following our plan, you'll be practiced enough to create your own meal plans going forward.

➤ **GOOGLE "WHOLE30 MEAL PLAN":** There are dozens of community-created meal planning resources available for free online. Just read your recipes carefully; these plans haven't been vetted by the Whole30 team, so we can't guarantee every recipe included is 100% compliant.

"I feel quite a bit of anxiety today. I thought I was prepared but then started doubting myself. A big part of me wants to say, 'Nah! Let's start Whole30 tomorrow.' But I know that I just have to start right here and right now, with no more excuses."

—*Tawnya D., Oregon*

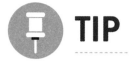

TIP

"No snacking" is just a general Whole30 *recommendation*, not a *rule*. As your body adapts, you'll learn how big to make your meals, how often you need to eat, and how to trust your body's hungry and full signals. But you're probably not there yet, and that's okay! It's smart to have snack options on hand this week, just in case. Make sure each snack includes protein, fat, or both. (A piece of fruit all by itself isn't very satiating, and the whole point of a snack is to get you from one meal to the next.) Try a hard-boiled egg with a handful of almonds, baby carrots with guacamole, or a meat stick and an apple. Eventually, you'll eliminate the need to snack on a regular basis—but know that if you're traveling, pregnant or nursing, feeding a growing kiddo, or having an especially active day, snacks *may* be necessary.

HACK

Habit experts say the key to staying motivated and feeling rewarded by your efforts is setting small mini-goals—achievable daily goals that give you the feeling of a "win" and take advantage of inertia (an object in motion stays in motion). If you're feeling overwhelmed at the idea of 30 WHOLE DAYS of this thing, stop and reframe. Your only goal? Just one day of Whole30. Eat Whole30 meals, sticking to the rules 100%, just for today. See that little box at the end of the day that says, "I did it?" THAT'S your goal. Small wins every day are how new, healthy habits are built—and you've already taken the first step.

EXTRA CREDIT: Create a thorough meal plan for tomorrow, using one of the strategies outlined here. Plan for breakfast, lunch, dinner, pre- and post-workout (if necessary), and emergency food (hard-boiled eggs, a meat stick, cashews, sliced veggies, an apple, a packet of almond butter, etc.) in case you need a snack.

Right now, you're thinking about food, snacks, more food . . . and survival. This is totally normal! You're still getting the hang of this Whole30 thing, and it gets easier with practice. It's also your first opportunity to reflect. Take the time to complete these sections thoughtfully; they've been carefully designed to keep you motivated, accountable, and seeing progress.

What went well today: _____

_____

_____

_____

_____

What could have gone better: _____

_____

_____

_____

_____

What I'll do tomorrow: _____

_____

_____

_____

_____

Today's Extra Credit: _____

_____

_____

_____

_____

_____

_____

Today's NSVs

Energy

The Worst   The Best!

1   2   3   4   5   6   7   8   9   10

NOTES: ....

....

Sleep Quality

The Worst   The Best!

1   2   3   4   5   6   7   8   9   10

NOTES: ....

....

Cravings

The Worst   The Best!

1   2   3   4   5   6   7   8   9   10

NOTES: ....

....

FILL IN YOUR OWN

NSV #1: ....

....

....

NSV #2: ....

....

....

NSV #3: ....

....

....

WHAT I ATE

Favorite!

☐ Meal 1: ....

....

....

☐ Meal 2: ....

....

....

☐ Meal 3: ....

....

....

Extra meal/snack: ....

....

....

Day 1 Reflections

....

....

....

....

....

....

☐ **I did it! Whole30 Day 1 is in the bag.**

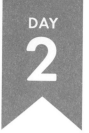

DAY 2

WELCOME TO DAY 2. Here's a virtual hug, because statistically, 94.3% of you are feeling headache-y, foggy, weak, slow, lightheaded, and lethargic. Welcome to The Hangover: no tequila required. This is where the ghosts of your high-carb past (cookies, chocolate, chips, ice cream, muffins, bread, wine) come back to kick you in the butt—or the head. The amount of suck you are feeling today is in direct proportion to the amount of junk you ate before your Whole30 began . . . anyone regretting their carb-a-palooza the night before Day 1? (In retrospect, "Let's just eat it all now so we're not tempted later" was not the best Whole30 preparatory strategy.)

The "hangover" is totally normal as your body starts to transition from running on sugar to being a fat-burning machine. The good news? It should only last a day or two—and some people skip it altogether. So pound some water, take it easy at the gym, and dim the lights . . . this too shall pass.

Melissa's Motivation

This part of your Whole30 generally isn't super fun. You're tired, hungry, missing the stuff you used to eat, and thinking, "This is *not* what I signed up for." Except it is. Even the hard parts. The sugar withdrawals, cravings, and challenges that come with learning how to relate to food in an entirely new way are evidence that something is changing. *You* are changing. And every time you yawn but keep going, crave and distract, feel hungry and feed yourself well, YOU WIN. And every tiny win adds up to HUGE changes.

A Whole30 reset is the jump-start to a *lifetime of food freedom*. Did you think that was gonna be easy? For most people, things get worse before they get better, and I want to be up front about that. But it *does* get better, easier, and more fun with practice. So be patient, be kind to yourself, and trust the process.

FAQ ◀━━━

I FEEL LIKE I'M STARVING ALL DAY LONG. Um, that's not really a question, but we feel you. It's really common to be hungry (like, brain-eating-zombie hungry) the first week on the program. Maybe you didn't plan for enough food, maybe you're a little fat-phobic, or maybe it's your brain staging a sugar rebellion, which feels a lot like hunger. Regardless, here are some tips.

→ **IF YOU HAVE TO SNACK, SNACK.** As we discussed yesterday, it's common to need a snack here and there as you figure out how much you need to eat at each meal. (Just don't graze mindlessly, m'kay?)

→ **PREPARE YOUR MEALS AND SNACKS,** but make sure you have extra food on hand just in case. Hard-boil a dozen eggs, have canned tuna in the pantry, or make a double batch of those meatballs in case your plan to eat three per meal needs a bump to four.

→ **ADD MORE FAT.** You've replaced calorie-dense carbs like bread, cereal, and pasta with lower-calorie veggies and fruit. Unless you pick up those calories somewhere else, you'll be under-eating. Confirm that you're eating at least a palm-sized serving of protein at each meal, then add a little more fat to help you feel satiated (like an extra slice of avocado, or an extra tablespoon of ghee on top of your roasted veggies).

COMMUNITY INSPIRATION

On easy ways to keep meals interesting: "At breakfast, we wanted a little something extra on top of our eggs and had to settle for jarred salsa. Today, I'm going to make a few fresh sauces out of my Whole30 books, for when our meals are little on the bland side."

—*Laura B.*

📌 TIP

You may not *want* to eat breakfast . . . but you really should. If your hormones (particularly leptin and cortisol) are out of whack based on what and when you used to eat, you may wake up feeling not that hungry—sometimes for hours. But waiting until 11 a.m. to eat "Meal 1" isn't going to help your cause! If you find you're just not hungry in the morning but *ravenous* after sundown, forcing yourself to eat a hearty, protein-rich breakfast will help you reset your appetite clock, and goes a long way toward beating p.m. cravings. It's okay to start off with a smaller meal as you get used to the idea, and breakfast doesn't have to contain tons of vegetables if that sounds icky. Just eat *something* well-balanced (protein, fat, and carbs), ideally within an hour of waking. Soon enough your appetite will catch up, and the kinds of foods you'll want to eat in the morning will expand.

HACK

Willpower is at its highest first thing in the morning, in part because sleep works miracles to replenish it. Why burn through any of it just thinking about what to cook for breakfast? (Yes, resisting the temptation to skip Meal 1 or pick up a technically-compliant-but-not-recommended fruit smoothie in favor of cooking a balanced meal DOES require willpower!) Today's habit hack is also tonight's Extra Credit: decide on breakfast *tonight*, so it's one less willpower-depleting decision for you to make tomorrow. Even better, prep your meal too, so even a Day-3-not-yet-caffeinated-crankypants-zombie can make it happen.

EXTRA CREDIT: Plan and prep tomorrow's breakfast—or better yet, a few days' worth of breakfasts! Make a dozen egg + veggie muffins, prep a frittata, or roast some vegetables and brown some breakfast sausage for easy reheating.

You might be feeling a little discouraged, or too tired to write down all of your feelings. Feel free to make it brief, use these pages to vent, or skip some sections entirely . . . but at a *bare minimum*: Do your Extra Credit (for which Future You will be grateful), document at least one NSV, and check off "I did it!" You've worked hard today, and that deserves recognition.

2

What went well today: ....

....

....

....

....

What could have gone better: ....

....

....

....

....

What I'll do tomorrow: ....

....

....

....

....

Today's Extra Credit:..

....

....

....

....

....

....

Today's NSVs

Energy

The Worst   The Best!

1   2   3   4   5   6   7   8   9   10

NOTES: ....

....

Sleep Quality

The Worst   The Best!

1   2   3   4   5   6   7   8   9   10

NOTES: ....

....

Cravings

The Worst   The Best!

1   2   3   4   5   6   7   8   9   10

NOTES: ....

....

FILL IN YOUR OWN

NSV #1: ....

....

....

NSV #2: ....

....

....

NSV #3: ....

....

....

WHAT I ATE

Favorite!

☐ Meal 1:..
....
....

☐ Meal 2:..
....
....

☐ Meal 3:..
....
....

Extra meal/snack:..
....
....

Day 2 Reflections

....
....
....
....
....
....

☐ **I did it! Whole30 Day 2 is in the bag.**

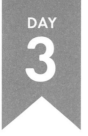

DAY 3

HELLO? HELLO! Sorry to wake you, just wanted to say, "Welcome to Day 3." This is a day of mixed emotions and physicality. You may be pumped one minute, discouraged the next. You may be energetic, then crash. You may have lingering headaches, or bathroom issues, or skin disruptions, or random cravings. And you're definitely wondering what the heck to do with yourself after dinner so you aren't prowling through the pantry.

Some of you may wake up thinking, "Huh. I actually feel pretty good." Yay for you! How good (or not good) you feel depends on a lot of things: health history, historical dietary patterns, activity level, stress levels . . . even the day you start can make a difference. (People who start on a weekend generally have a tougher time than those who start on a weekday, where routine is more firmly in place and temptations aren't as variable.) Just accept where you are now, and know it's all building up to the magic that is to come.

Melissa's Motivation

Sometimes, being told what to do is appreciated more than a peppy rah-rah speech, so . . . First, wherever you are, *it's normal.* (Probably. See the FAQ.) Don't worry about whether or not you're doing the "perfect" Whole30. Are you following the rules 100%? Then you're doing it right.

Second, if you're hungry, *go eat something.* Snack if you have to. Make sure each snack has protein, fat, or both. An apple all by itself is not a snack; it's a recipe for additional sugar cravings and more hunger 20 minutes after you finish it.

Finally, SLEEP. Go to bed early, even if it means you're not current with *The Walking Dead*/Facebook/Twitter/Instagram/email/ your sister's dating recap/Lego cleanup. Your body is working HARD, and willpower is replenished tremendously when we sleep. Future You will thank you for the extra hour.

FAQ

I FEEL A, B, AND C, BUT DON'T FEEL D. IS THIS NORMAL?
The Whole30 Timeline is a tongue-in-cheek but pretty darn accurate estimation of how you're feeling on any given day, but some days it's easier to draw conclusions than others, and as always, your mileage may vary. If you skip a stage, find yourself "off" by a few days, or experience something we haven't talked about, that doesn't mean you're doing anything wrong! However, the tendency is to blame *everything* on the Whole30. Flat tire/bad hair day/tingles in my pinkie finger? Must be a Whole30 side effect. Of course, not *everything* is Whole30-related. Here's a rough guide to what's normal . . . and what isn't.

NORMAL: Digestive distress (constipation, bloating, diarrhea), fatigue, headaches, sleepiness, fogginess, crankiness, cravings, breakouts. Also, if you have a chronic health condition (like fatigue) or autoimmune condition (like rheumatoid arthritis), it's possible that your usual symptoms will get worse before they get better.

NOT NORMAL: Nausea, vomiting, abdominal pain, vertigo or dizziness, fainting, rashes or hives, sinus congestion, runny nose, coughing, or fever. If you have any of these symptoms, please see your doctor. It's entirely possible you're dealing with seasonal allergies, the common cold, food poisoning, or a flu or virus.

"I've learned after five Whole30s to give myself some grace in the first few days, snack when needed so I don't get hangry, and nap or go to bed early. I also resist jumping into a new workout routine, just taking it easy and going for walks. The first few days are no joke!" —*Jaime B., Colorado*

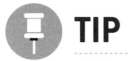

TIP

Your lethargy, crankiness, or lack of motivation may also mean you're just trying to do too much. Attempting high-intensity workouts or long runs, staying up late to do one more load of laundry, or refusing to snack even when you're starving can make your symptoms worse! You may also be trying to business-travel, nurse a baby, recover from an injury, or deal with some form of psychological stress, all of which will impact how this adjustment period goes. The first week of the Whole30 is tough, so take a rest or half-intensity day: skip basically everything in favor of bed, practice lots of healthy self-care, and for the sake of you *and* everyone around you, just eat the darn snack.

HACK

Attentional bias describes our tendency to pay attention to some things while ignoring others. When you're immersed in the Whole30, it's easy to think *everything* is Whole30-related. You'll overlook the fact that it's April, the trees are in bloom, and pollen is everywhere . . . and assume your sneezing and itchy eyes are a Whole30 side effect. If you're experiencing something "off" or negative, look at *all* your inputs. Are you under-slept, over-worked, or is it flu season? If you're having trouble stepping out of the bias to evaluate, ask someone not on the Whole30 to help you problem-solve. Also know this bias can be of benefit! Since you've got Whole30 on the brain, you'll be hyper-aware of food cues ("Donuts in the break room!"), which helps you manage them.

EXTRA CREDIT: Write down a few areas of your life *besides* your diet that may be contributing to stress, lethargy, or other negative symptoms, and create a plan for managing them. And if you feel awesome, write down a few things in your life besides the Whole30 that are contributing to that, too!

Today, search for all of the good things you already see happening as the result of your Whole30 journey—even if your Negative Nancy brain thinks you'll have to search *hard*. You may be tired, grumpy, or bloated, but you've seen some small wins today. Document them in each section of today's reflections, as a reminder that even better days are ahead!

What went well today: ....

What could have gone better: ....

What I'll do tomorrow: ....

Today's Extra Credit: ....

3

Today's NSVs

Energy

The Worst   The Best!

1   2   3   4   5   6   7   8   9   10

NOTES: ....

....

Sleep Quality

The Worst   The Best!

1   2   3   4   5   6   7   8   9   10

NOTES: ....

....

Cravings

The Worst   The Best!

1   2   3   4   5   6   7   8   9   10

NOTES: ....

....

FILL IN YOUR OWN

NSV #1: ....

....

....

NSV #2: ....

....

....

NSV #3: ....

....

....

WHAT I ATE

Favorite!

☐ Meal 1: ....
....
....

☐ Meal 2: ....
....
....

☐ Meal 3: ....
....
....

Extra meal/snack: ....
....
....

3

Day 3 Reflections

....
....
....
....
....
....

☐ **I did it! Whole30 Day 3 is in the bag.**

DAY 4 DAWNS and you tentatively step out of bed, wondering what this day will bring. Your brain is surprisingly clear. Your limbs all feel functional. This could be a good day! You walk into the kitchen, see the smiling faces of your beloved family . . . and have the sudden desire to punch them in the face. Welcome to the most famous Whole30 stage: Kill All the Things (KATT).

Your brain doesn't like being told "no," and it's gone THREE WHOLE DAYS without chocolate/diet soda/wine/chips. Throw in blood sugar dysregulation, disturbed sleep, and digestive distress—and it's no wonder you're cranky. This is also often accompanied by KATT's cousin Eat All the Things, where you're hungry all the time *how is this possible I JUST ATE*.

This, too, shall pass. Keep a low profile, take a deep breath, and remember why you started the Whole30 in the first place. This usually lasts no more than a day or two . . . but your spouse *really* hopes it's just one.

Melissa's Motivation

Our Timeline doesn't always predict sunshine, rainbows, and ponies, but that doesn't mean you should start your day with trepidation. We're up front about potential negatives just in case you *do* wake up feeling off. But there is benefit in keeping a positive mindset and expecting the best out of the experience.

Your headache, lethargy, or digestive distress may be real, but you can choose how you respond to it. Don't wake up *expecting* to feel like poop; instead, start your day with, "I'm one day closer to Tiger Blood!" If you find yourself feeling less-than-awesome, actively seek out the positives you're already seeing. And if you're feeling better than the Timeline predicted, celebrate! Your mind is a powerful thing, and thinking you're going to breeze through your Whole30 goes a long way toward you breezing through your Whole30.

FAQ ◀──

HOW AM I SUPPOSED TO GET THROUGH 26 MORE DAYS OF THIS? It's normal to want to look ahead, anticipating how great you'll feel when your 30 days are up. But it can also be paralyzing to think about *so many more days* of meal prep, dishes, resisting temptation, and social challenges, especially when you're already feeling tired, bloated, cranky, and craving. Your strategy: "One day at a time."

──▶ We warned you on page 22 that looking way down the road at a long-term goal can be daunting and demotivating. Instead, we encouraged you to set achievable goals, allowing you to feel the satisfaction of regular rewards instead of waiting days and days for the "payoff." On the Whole30, your mini-goal is completing just one day of the program, 100% by the books.

──▶ Some days, however, even *this* will feel hard. Stressful days, restless nights, and unplanned challenges can leave you feeling ready to bail. Here, you're best served by breaking your goal down even further; just focus on making your next *meal* Whole30 compliant. That's it; just one meal. You can do that! When that meal is done (and you're surely feeling better), give yourself a high-five for sticking to your commitment . . . and repeat.

> COMMUNITY INSPIRATION
>
> "I've been working on my word choices. Moving from 'I can't eat that' to 'I choose not to.' And I'm not 'on a diet,' I'm on 'a program leading me toward a healthier lifestyle.' I realize every word, whether positive or negative, will affect my progress." —*Jeannette W., Illinois*

4

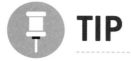

TIP

Today would be a great day to be proactive in changing your habits, giving you a real sense of accomplishment to counteract your KATT symptoms. Kill two birds with one stone by creating a new nighttime routine to replace your *old* routine of frantically prowling through the pantry looking for something saltyfatty-sweetcrunchy. And no, it shouldn't involve technically-compliant Whole30 sweet stuff, so back away from serving up a dried-fruit-and-nut bar on your best china. Brew a pot of herbal tea and sit down with a good book, draw yourself a bath, lay out your gym clothes and prep for breakfast, or up your dental game and do a long floss/electric brush/rinse routine. (Bonus: this sends a strong signal that "eating time is over"—buh-bye cravings!)

HACK

Habit research shows having physical representation of your progress toward a goal keeps you more motivated, accountable, and on track than a mental checkbox. (Why do you think there's a box for you to check off at the end of every day?) If you're a super-visual person or want your accountability even more front-and-center, mount a calendar on the wall, fill one mason jar with 30 stones and place an empty one next to it, or create a colorful paper chain with an affirmation written on each one. Then at the end of every day, make an "X" on your calendar, move a stone from one jar to the other, or remove one link from the chain to mark your progress.

EXTRA CREDIT: Do *one thing* before you go to bed to prep for the coming day—something that will have a big payoff in the morning. Wash all the dishes so you wake to a spotless kitchen; prep breakfast AND lunch; or write yourself a love note of encouragement and post it on the bathroom mirror. Then, go to bed early. That's an order.

Today is all about showing yourself grace for the ups and the downs you may be experiencing at this stage in your Whole30 journey. Remind yourself that wherever you are, you're succeeding, and are exactly where you should be in the process. Use positive words and messaging in today's reflections, and take EXTRA satisfaction in checking off the "I did it" box!

What went well today: ....

....

....

....

....

What could have gone better: ....

....

....

....

....

What I'll do tomorrow: ....

....

....

....

....

Today's Extra Credit: ....

....

....

....

....

....

....

....

4

Today's NSVs

Energy

The Worst   The Best!

1   2   3   4   5   6   7   8   9   10

NOTES: ....

....

Sleep Quality

The Worst   The Best!

1   2   3   4   5   6   7   8   9   10

NOTES: ....

....

Cravings

The Worst   The Best!

1   2   3   4   5   6   7   8   9   10

NOTES: ....

....

FILL IN YOUR OWN

NSV #1: ....

....

....

NSV #2: ....

....

....

NSV #3: ....

....

....

WHAT I ATE

Favorite!

☐ Meal 1: ....
....
....

☐ Meal 2: ....
....
....

☐ Meal 3: ....
....

Extra meal/snack: ....
....
....

4

Day 4 Reflections

....
....
....
....
....
....
....

☐ **I did it! Whole30 Day 4 is in the bag.**

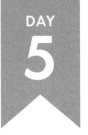

DAY 5

DAY 5 IS A MIXED BAG . . . and if you immediately thought "bag of potato chips," you're not alone. Your KATT may still be lingering, but even if you're less cranky, you could be feeling more anxious and unsure. Week 1 can make you feel like you're a ship being tossed around by a storm, so today is all about settling in with some practical advice to keep you feeling anchored and not so "motion sick."

If you're still tired, ravenously hungry (or not at all hungry), cranky, moody, or feeling impatient, this is normal. Your body and brain are still settling into this new routine, and it's only been five days—even if it feels like much longer. If you're starting to get a glimpse of the sun through the storm clouds, take heart! Be happy with the bursts of energy, clarity, and NSVs, even if they don't last all day. They're a sign that your ship is moving in the right direction.

Melissa's Motivation

You're dedicated to the Whole30 rules; following our recommendations, planning your meals, and distracting your way through temptations. But please, don't try to do the "perfect" Whole30. First, because it doesn't exist. Not every meal will fit our template, not every ingredient will be hand-made with love, and at least once, you'll skip dinner and just go to bed because *please let this day end.* Also, the Whole30 is just the first step toward a *lifetime* of practicing your food freedom! You don't have to figure it all out in 30 days.

Still hungry between meals? Eat a snack! Gave into dessert cravings with an apple and almond butter? Acknowledge this is a habit you're working on, but know that *you stayed Whole30 compliant*, and that's a huge win! Remember, your goal is to complete the Whole30 exactly as written for 30 straight days. And checking five "I did it!" boxes in a row is gold-star-worthy all by itself.

FAQ

HOW DO I KNOW IF I'M EATING TOO MUCH? If you're used to logging every bite, it can be scary to drop the calorie-counting, macro-tracking, or food-measuring, but people are more likely to *under*eat than overeat on the Whole30!

→ You've replaced calorie-dense grains, beans, and processed foods with veggies and fruits, and upped your healthy fats to fill in the gap. But if you're still fat-phobic and/or hyper-focused on weight loss, you may not be adding enough. The fat recommendations in our meal template (page 6) are a *minimum* per meal . . . don't go below, or your metabolism will start working against you.

→ The foods you're eating (with complete protein, natural fats, and lots of micronutrients) are way more satiating than the processed foods you used to eat, which means you'll feel full faster. This can prompt people to skip lunch or eat really small meals, which can lead to being underfed. Three meals a day following our template is, again, the minimum you should be aiming for.

NOTE: The meal template will keep you in the right ballpark, but you should also be adjusting each meal size based on hunger, energy, and athletic performance. If two weeks in, you're still constantly hungry, lethargic, and foggy, eat more!

> **COMMUNITY INSPIRATION**
>
> "This morning I have so much energy! I actually wondered, *Is there Tiger Blood in my veins?* We'll see if it lasts, because midday and last night I was soooo tired. I am also noticing changes in my physical appearance. Feeling hopeful!"
>
> —*Elizabeth M., Colorado*

📌 TIP

You may be struggling with the temptation of having "just a sip/bite/taste" of non-compliant food. Who would know, and what will it *really* hurt? First, YOU would know. You made a commitment to yourself: 30 days of 100% Whole30. How will it make you feel to sneak around the rules? Is that bite of pizza really worth breaking your commitment? The guilt or hit to your self-confidence might even spiral you into more poor food choices. Plus, just one sip/bite will break the "reset" you're trying to achieve with 30 days of strict elimination! Remind yourself that you've been here before, and caving to momentary temptation just isn't worth it. Five minutes later, you'll be happy you stuck it out.

HACK

When I counsel recovering addicts who are tempted to use, I offer one rule: You have to tell someone first—connecting in person, via phone or text, or chat (no voicemails!)—and you must open with "I am planning to use and abandon my recovery." The strategy has proven incredibly successful—the very idea of the conversation may make the urge disappear, but even if it doesn't, this scripted moment of pause between craving and reward is huge in reducing the urge. You can use this during your Whole30, when you're tempted to have "just one bite." Before you do, you have to tell your Whole30 support group, best friend, or mom, "I'm about to break my Whole30 for a bite of chips and salsa," and wait for a response *before* you take that bite. Trust me, if willpower fails . . . this will not.

EXTRA CREDIT: Secure a few Whole30 buddies you can count on day or night if you really get stuck and need help. Ask them, "If I run into a tight Whole30 spot, can I text you for encouragement?" Keep the list of people nearby, and don't be afraid to use it!

Now that you know you don't have to do the "perfect Whole30" (whew!), you should have a little extra capacity and generosity to document all of the awesome things you have been doing, saying, thinking, and feeling over the last five days. Cram those NSVs in today, no matter how small, and remind yourself that you are worth the commitment.

What went well today: ....

....

....

....

....

What could have gone better: ....

....

....

....

What I'll do tomorrow: ....

....

....

....

Today's Extra Credit: ....

....

....

....

....

....

5

Today's NSVs

Energy

The Worst | | | | | | | | | The Best!

1 2 3 4 5 6 7 8 9 10

NOTES: ....

....

Sleep Quality

The Worst | | | | | | | | | The Best!

1 2 3 4 5 6 7 8 9 10

NOTES: ....

....

Cravings

The Worst | | | | | | | | | The Best!

1 2 3 4 5 6 7 8 9 10

NOTES: ....

....

FILL IN YOUR OWN

NSV #1: ....

....

....

NSV #2: ....

....

....

NSV #3: ....

....

....

WHAT I ATE

Favorite!

☐ Meal 1: ....
....
....

☐ Meal 2: ....
....
....

☐ Meal 3: ....
....

Extra meal/snack: ....
....
....

5

Day 5 Reflections

....
....
....
....
....
....

☐ **I did it! Whole30 Day 5 is in the bag.**

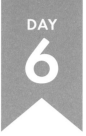

DAY 6

DAY 6 might be another roller coaster of a ride. You feel awesome! You're exhausted. You're starving! Nothing sounds good. You're so sleepy! You toss and turn. Sounds a lot like Day 5, but there's one difference...Day 6 tends to be a breakthrough day, as in the coming days, you'll *finally* crest the top of the track and start flying down with your hands in the air.

Your body is working hard to catch up to your new healthy habits, but you can't just flip a switch and restore a healthy balance. Today is all about the science, because for many people, knowing *why* you're feeling this way helps you feel less anxious and more forgiving of your body and brain for all the ups and downs. Stay focused on the positives, get excited when you see evidence of the progress you've been working so hard for, and know that better days are just around the corner... wheeeee!

Melissa's Motivation

Today, remind yourself *why* you're doing the Whole30, or dig back into the science behind the program to shore up your motivational foundation. You really miss your a.m. carbs ... why can't you make pancakes, again? (See page 95 in *The Whole30*.) You're dying to step on the scale—but doesn't the scale hold you hostage, your self-confidence hanging in the balance? (Google "Whole30 5 Reasons to Ditch the Scale" for reinforcement.) Your cravings are persistent ... are you doing something wrong? (Nope; it's the processed foods you used to eat, and the effect of chronic stress. See Chapter 4 in *It Starts With Food*, and watch my "Stress and Cravings" video at w30.co/mh-stress-cravings.

Finally, remind yourself where you started, and compare it to where you are today. Bare minimum, you're six days closer to food freedom, and that alone should be motivating!

FAQ

WHAT'S HAPPENING IN MY BODY? The first week on the Whole30 can be rough, but it helps to know what's going on "under the hood." Many of your symptoms this week have to do with fat adaptation.

> Your body is used to running on sugar for fuel, thanks to all the grains, added sugar, and processed carbs you used to eat. But on a low-sugar Whole30 diet, your body isn't getting the "gas" it needs. It's like a car sputtering on an empty tank, looking for a quick and easy fill-up. (Carb cravings, anyone?) Now, there's another energy source just sitting there, ready to be tapped into . . . fat! If you could do that, you'd be like a hybrid, cruising steadily on electricity (fat) but still able to step on the gas (glucose) when you need quick energy.

> The fat adaptation process starts in just a few days, but takes a few weeks to fully ramp up. Right now, you're stuck in no-man's-land . . . running on fumes, with the charging station still a few days down the road. THIS is why you have headaches, lethargy, sleepiness, fogginess, cravings, and unusual hunger. Your body is looking for the energy source it *used* to run on, not quite able to tap into the energy source you've already got plenty of. The good news? Keep eating your Whole30 meals, naturally low in sugar with plenty of healthy fats, and your body *will* cruise into the Tiger Blood charging station!

6

"I think we are going to have to start going to sleep immediately following dinner to prevent these overgrown hunger spells . . . BUT as I sit here and write, I'm starting to get that Whole30 energy shot running through me."   —*Kirk H., California*

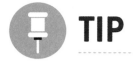 **TIP**

Kirk H. was *mostly* kidding, but lots of Whole30ers at this stage confess to climbing into bed early as a last-ditch effort to combat p.m. cravings, reset a cranky mood, recover from their attempted workout, and promote good energy levels in the morning. While it may seem like a moment of desperation to turn in at 8 p.m., it's actually not a bad idea. How many times can we say, "Your body is working hard" here? Giving it a little more rest will help you heal, recover, and reset faster, and make you feel like a healthy-living rock star when you wake up after 9 solid hours. Plus, nothing good happens (in your kitchen) between the hours of 8 p.m. and midnight anyway. (You know this is true.)

HACK

Another benefit of sleeping more? A full willpower tank come morning. A 2015 neuroscience study found that sleep-deprived individuals are more likely to give in to impulses, have less focus, and don't have as much energy to exercise willpower. Those who sleep more (or take naps), however, are more likely to stick to a goal even when frustrated, and report feeling less impulsive. Not getting enough sleep is also stressful, and as you learned in my YouTube talk from the Motivation section (page 50), stress promotes cravings. Isn't that a double-edged sword? When you skimp on sleep, you crave more sugar *and* have less willpower—lose/lose. We'll talk about sleep in more detail on Day 18, but the summary is found in today's Extra Credit.

EXTRA CREDIT: Go to bed early. Like, guilty-pleasure-early. Toddler-early. If you feel weird about this, climb into bed with a book (a real book, not an e-reader) and a mug of herbal tea and read for a while—but no TV, smartphone, or stressful discussions. Your willpower, energy, and mood will thank you tomorrow.

Are you getting excited, knowing what's just around the corner? Even if today was tough, take the time to note the positives, and choose to see the energy, sleep, or craving struggles as signs of progress. Your body, brain, habits, and relationship with food are all changing for the better, and after a good night's sleep, your Whole30 will look bright and shiny again.

What went well today: ....

....

....

....

....

What could have gone better: ....

....

....

....

What I'll do tomorrow: ....

....

....

....

Today's Extra Credit:...

....

....

....

....

....

....

6

Today's NSVs

Energy

The Worst   The Best!

1   2   3   4   5   6   7   8   9   10

NOTES: ....

....

Sleep Quality

The Worst   The Best!

1   2   3   4   5   6   7   8   9   10

NOTES: ....

....

Cravings

The Worst   The Best!

1   2   3   4   5   6   7   8   9   10

NOTES: ....

....

FILL IN YOUR OWN

NSV #1: ....

....

....

NSV #2: ....

....

....

NSV #3: ....

....

....

WHAT I ATE

Favorite!

☐ Meal 1: ....
....
....

☐ Meal 2: ....
....
....

☐ Meal 3: ....
....
....

Extra meal/snack: ....
....
....

6

Day 6 Reflections

....
....
....
....
....
....
....

☐ **I did it! Whole30 Day 6 is in the bag.**

DAY 7 = ONE WEEK of Whole30! While you feel like you're past the worst of it, you may also have some anxiety. It's common to wonder, "What if it's not working?" It's tempting to think, "I should check the scale to make *sure* it's working." Maybe you're even discouraged; "I thought I'd be further along than this . . . shouldn't I be seeing more changes by now?"

This is normal, given your history with dieting. It's been beaten into your head that for a diet to "work," you have to restrict, be hungry, and put your willpower to the test every second of every day. Heck, it's almost like being miserable on a diet is a badge of honor. And here, well, you're just not! You're eating delicious food. You're not starving. Your meals are satiating. And you're already seeing improvements! So instead of anxiety, decide that today is a day to feel *hopeful*. Keep reading, trust the process, and get excited for what's to come.

Melissa's Motivation

You're eating full meals. You're not counting, weighing, measuring, or feeling deprived (though you might miss bread). So . . . how can this be working? Because the Whole30 isn't a *diet*; it's a *reset*. Taste buds, blood sugar regulation, hormones, digestion, and your immune system are all returning to a healthy balance. You're resetting emotionally, too, learning a new language around food, changing your habits, and creating awareness of how the foods you used to eat were impacting your self-confidence, motivation, and quality of life.

If this feels different, that's because it IS different. (And that's a good thing, because all those other diets didn't end up working very well.) The Whole30 has changed the lives of millions of people, and looking back through six days of reflections, it's clear to see that it IS already working for you. Carry on!

FAQ

WHY CAN'T I TRACK OR COUNT? While not a rule, "tracking" (entering foods, quantities, and analyzing or planning to consume the caloric or macronutrient results) is *seriously* discouraged on the Whole30.

→ Tracking may hold you back from the very thing you're hoping to achieve—getting back in touch with your body's natural regulatory mechanisms, trusting your hunger, and knowing when to stop eating. During your Whole30, these signals will actually start to work, perhaps for the first time in years—and we want you to be guided by them, because your body knows how much you should be eating better than any internet calculator.

→ We've designed our meal template (page 6) with healthy, sustainable weight loss built right in . . . but some of you have been so conditioned to restrict that even though you feel amazing, you may still be tempted to cut back once you see the numbers add up. That could spell big trouble for your metabolism, as you can easily end up undereating!

→ Skipping the weighing, measuring, and tracking will help you foster a healthier relationship with food and turn mealtime into a relaxing, enjoyable experience instead of a complicated math session. So use these 30 days to break the habit and truly reconnect with your body—because no one ever found *true* food freedom being chained to a tracking app.

COMMUNITY INSPIRATION

"This is my fourth Whole30. To people struggling . . . trust the program and the process. As your body relearns to do what it is meant to, your health (and your waistline) *will* improve. Look for the NSVs and just take it one meal at a time. If I can do this, you can do this."   —*Terry G., British Columbia*

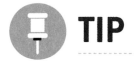
TIP

It's been a whole week, and you really want to jump on the scale to see how far you've come. But remember, you're here for so much more than weight loss! (And the scale won't reflect all of the positive results you're seeing—which may leave you with *less* resolve.) You have so many other ways to measure your Whole30 success (NSVs), and some of them are physical. Are your rings, shirts, or pants fitting better? Is your skin clearer, are your joints less swollen, is your nose less stuffy? Practice relying on something *other* than scale weight to help you stay motivated and on track, and pretty soon you'll realize it doesn't matter what the scale says when it comes to your health and happiness.

HACK

Psychologist BJ Fogg says that sticking with good habits is less about creating motivation, and more about *taking advantage* of motivation when you have it. As different people are inspired by different things, and inspiration hits us at different times of day, the hard part is *noticing* that you're feeling energetic. So the next time you catch yourself feeling especially driven, ride that "motivational wave" to do the hard things you've been thinking about doing but still haven't done. Delete the food tracking app from your phone, donate your scale to charity, or get rid of the "just in case" chocolate from your pantry. Take advantage when you're feeling strong to protect Future You when things get tough.

EXTRA CREDIT: Identify time periods today when you felt super motivated—ready to tackle food prep, hard conversations, or challenging temptations. Write down the circumstances; did you have a good night's sleep, a great meal, or notice a new NSV? Identify trends, so you can be on the lookout for (or create!) high-motivation periods ahead.

Today is all about realizing you are *not* your numbers—calories, scale weight, or grams of carbs—and embracing this new way of thinking about food, health, and your body. The Whole30 is so different from anything you've ever done before, and it's okay to feel unsure . . . so use today's reflection space to counteract that by identifying all of the ways it's *already* working for you.

What went well today: ....

....

....

....

....

What could have gone better: ....

....

....

....

....

What I'll do tomorrow: ....

....

....

....

....

Today's Extra Credit:..

....

....

....

....

....

....

....

Today's NSVs

Energy

The Worst   The Best!

1   2   3   4   5   6   7   8   9   10

NOTES: ....

....

Sleep Quality

The Worst   The Best!

1   2   3   4   5   6   7   8   9   10

NOTES: ....

....

Cravings

The Worst   The Best!

1   2   3   4   5   6   7   8   9   10

NOTES: ....

....

FILL IN YOUR OWN

NSV #1: ....

....

....

NSV #2: ....

....

....

NSV #3: ....

....

....

WHAT I ATE

Favorite!

☐ Meal 1: ....
....
....
....

☐ Meal 2: ....
....
....
....

☐ Meal 3: ....
....
....
....

Extra meal/snack: ....
....
....

Day 7 Reflections

....
....
....
....
....
....
....

☐ **I did it! Whole30 Day 7 is in the bag.**

DAY 8

HAPPY DAY 8! Things are *finally* starting to feel like they're clicking . . . until your Sugar Dragon rears his ugly head. During the first week, it's actually easier to resist cravings; the program is exciting and willpower is high. But rolling into week two (and not quite feeling the magic yet), you may start seeing temptation around every corner.

We've been preparing you for this for the last few days; reminding you of all the ways your Whole30 IS working so when the sugar starts calling, you'll be firm in your resolve. But don't panic if you're still having cravings. Your habits and emotions are still catching up with your new food choices, putting you in tough spots *without* allowing you the usual sweets and treats as crutches. It may feel like you're white-knuckling it past every temptation, but it will get easier as your taste buds change, blood sugar regulates, and you develop new healthy habits. In the meantime, use our tips to see you through.

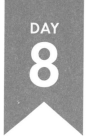 ## Melissa's Motivation

Today's motivation comes with a healthy dose of tough love: The easiest way to keep cravings at bay is to avoid temptation in the first place. "Duh," you say, but how often are you thinking about cravings *before* they happen? Chances are, you're only aware of the craving once it hits you like an 18-wheeler, and you're left scrambling to handle it in a way that doesn't involve tackling your donut-bearing co-worker to the ground.

The habit research term is called "pre-commitment": limiting your choices while you're in a safe space away from temptation. It's telling the waiter not to bring the dessert menu, or avoiding the break room leftovers after a birthday party. Don't be fearful or obsessive—just think ahead, and give yourself a planned "out" where you can, increasing your self-confidence and willpower for future temptations.

FAQ

HOW DO I KNOW IF I'M HUNGRY OR JUST HAVING A CRAVING? It's not always easy to tell the difference, especially in the heat of the moment with temptation staring you in the face. Here are two methods to help you figure out whether your body just needs to eat something hearty and healthy, or if it's just your Sugar Dragon breathing fire.

> **HALT:** This acronym stands for Hungry, Angry, Lonely, Tired. The next time you're having a craving, stop and ask yourself, "Am I really hungry, or am I just angry, lonely, or tired . . . or anxious, bored, frustrated, in pain . . . ," you get the picture. If you can honestly assess that you're not really hungry, distract yourself for a few minutes to see you through. If the self-assessment helps you realize you really *are* hungry, then eat a full meal or a mini-meal to tide you over (see Hack).

> **STEAMED FISH AND BROCCOLI:** This next trick is a bit simpler, but brutally effective. Just ask yourself, "Am I hungry enough to eat steamed fish and broccoli right now?" (Or hard-boiled eggs and guacamole, or plain roasted chicken with carrot sticks.) If the answer is, "No, but I'd eat an RxBar or some grapes . . ." then you're just craving, so distract yourself accordingly. If the answer is "Yes," then you really *are* hungry. (But you don't have to eat steamed fish and broccoli —any mini-meal will do.)

8

COMMUNITY INSPIRATION

"This weekend was soooo hard . . . BUT I MADE IT!!!! I wrote a big long post in the Whole30 Forum all about my cravings while I was having them, which kept me occupied long enough that I lost the craving edge and just decided to go to bed. I'm proud of myself!!" —*Christina C., Kent, UK*

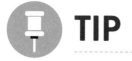

TIP

According to willpower research (done with smokers), the average craving lasts just 3 to 5 minutes. And according to *other* willpower research (done with toddlers and marshmallows), the best way to resist a craving is with distraction. So if you failed the Steamed Fish and Broccoli Test, do a few sun salutations, pay a bill, wash the dishes, tidy your desk, fold the laundry, chat with a friend, scroll through an inspirational Instagram feed, or read a few pages of your book. Giving your brain a break from the immediacy of the reward will help you prioritize your long-term goal of completing the Whole30 over immediate (but short-lived) gratification. Before you know it, your craving will be buh-bye, and your Sugar Dragon will be one step closer to snoozin' in his cave.

HACK

If you've got a sweet tooth at mealtime, you might be tempted to satisfy it with something sweet-but-compliant, like dates or a dried-fruit-and-nut bar. After all, it's not as bad as a chocolate bar, right? Resist—that's the *worst* thing you could do! Your brain doesn't know the difference between a Snickers bar and a Larabar, it just knows "I craved sugar, and I got sugar!" The perfect craving-busting meal or snack shouldn't include anything that could fire up your Sugar Dragon, so fill your plate with something savory and satisfying, based on protein, healthy fat, and veggies. Note, the same rule applies for mini-meals. (A banana alone is not a good snack!)

EXTRA CREDIT: Write down some temptations you've experienced so far in your Whole30 journey, and least one way you could have avoided them. (Hint: if the temptation came from your own pantry; it's time to clean out your pantry. For real this time.) This will cut your potential for craving encounters down substantially!

One of the best distractions for craving is journaling. You don't have to wait until the end of your Whole30 day to share your reflections, make if/then plans, or track your NSVs. The next time you feel a craving hit, grab this book and scribble away. You'll both tame your Sugar Dragon *and* make valuable observations to use during the rest of your Whole30. Win/win!

What went well today: ....

....

....

....

....

What could have gone better: ....

....

....

....

What I'll do tomorrow: ....

....

....

....

Today's Extra Credit: ....

....

....

....

....

....

....

8

Today's NSVs

Energy

The Worst   The Best!

1   2   3   4   5   6   7   8   9   10

NOTES: ....

....

Sleep Quality

The Worst   The Best!

1   2   3   4   5   6   7   8   9   10

NOTES: ....

....

Cravings

The Worst   The Best!

1   2   3   4   5   6   7   8   9   10

NOTES: ....

....

FILL IN YOUR OWN

NSV #1: ....

....

....

NSV #2: ....

....

....

NSV #3: ....

....

....

WHAT I ATE

Favorite!

☐ Meal 1:...
....
....
....

☐ Meal 2:...
....
....
....

☐ Meal 3:...
....
....
....

Extra meal/snack:...
....
....

Day 8 Reflections

....
....
....
....
....
....

8

☐ **I did it! Whole30 Day 8 is in the bag.**

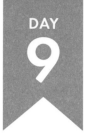

DAY

9

WELCOME TO DAY 9 . . . the "Food Day." At this point in your Whole30 journey, it seems like all you're doing is thinking about food. Planning food. Chopping food. Cleaning up after food. Looking at other people's food. Talking about your food. Maybe even dreaming about food. You may be tired of what you've been eating (eggs on eggs on eggs). You may be irrationally frustrated with other people who "get to eat whatever they want." You may be tired of people asking you about this "crazy diet" you're on. We get it . . . but it won't always be like this.

Any new behavior demands that you pay attention to the details until the actions become habit. When you first started driving, it was "seat belt, mirrors, signal, what gear am I in?" But as driving felt more familiar, you were able to pull back from the minutiae and enjoy the scenery. Same here. You won't always be thinking so much about the food, but for now (while you're learning), here are some tips.

Melissa's Motivation

It may seem like the Whole30 has taken over your whole life, but that's only because you're forming new habits—the hardest part of this journey. Your brain's executive function is in overdrive, making decisions about what to do when you crave, what to order instead of tacos, and what to say when someone asks about your lunch. But practice makes perfect, and you've had nine days of practice!

Think about Day 1, when you felt unsure about just about *everything*. Compare that to yesterday, when you effortlessly packed a lunch, grabbed a meat stick when the meeting ran late, and went straight to the tea cabinet instead of the pantry after dinner. You've already created some new habits, so don't sweat how hard you're still working in other areas. Soon enough, you'll be effortlessly cruising down the Whole30 highway.

FAQ ◀━━━

HOW DO I RESPOND WHEN PEOPLE ASK ME ABOUT MY "CRAZY DIET"? If the Whole30 is a radical departure from the way you used to eat or lots of your social engagements center around food or alcohol, it's natural for people to be curious about your new "diet." The key is being prepared, and practicing your responses to commonly asked questions.

━━▶ REFINE YOUR "ELEVATOR PITCH." Building on page 15, expand your description of the Whole30. Keep it positive, avoid negative buzzwords like "diet" or "cleanse," and share your personal reasons for doing it. "I've been exhausted, my shoulder still hurts, and my sugar cravings are out of control, so I'm doing a 30-day reset designed to help me figure out which foods might be contributing to the problem. I eliminate a bunch of stuff for 30 days, then reintroduce it and see how it impacts me. So far I'm feeling great, I'm never hungry, and the food I'm eating is delicious."

━━▶ PRACTICE MAKES PERFECT. Then, practice your pitch! The more effortlessly this rolls off your tongue, the more sure of yourself you'll sound when explaining it, and the less you'll be inviting criticism, skepticism, or peer pressure to "have just one." Make it clear with a confident tone and bright smile that your food choices are not up for debate, then change the subject to something *not* food-related.

COMMUNITY INSPIRATION

"If people try to push food on you in social situations . . . just say 'no thank you' and change the subject. It doesn't matter why or why not. You choose not to eat it, and everyone else needs to respect that, because that's how adults treat other adults." —@notacommittee

9

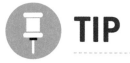

TIP

Have you figured out ways to make this "eating real food" and "cooking at home" thing easier? Maybe it's preparing double batches of everything. Maybe it's buying pre-chopped or spiralized veggies, or Whole30 Approved salad dressings and mayo. Or maybe it's realizing that not every Whole30 meal has to be a religious experience, and it's okay if dinner is grass-fed hot dogs, store-bought applesauce, and leftover veggies. If you discover a shortcut that lets you stick to the Whole30 in a satisfying, compliant way, *take it when you need it*. Remember, if you want to turn this into a lifestyle, it has to be sustainable! But that's not an excuse to eat a meat stick for breakfast three mornings in a row because you're too lazy to cook. Shortcuts are helpful, but if you want to make the most of your Whole30, you've still gotta put in the effort, people.

HACK

Habit research shows it's hard to start a new behavior, but once you get started, the tendency of an object in motion to stay in motion works in your favor. However, people can spend *so* much energy on the "getting started" part that they struggle to sustain the change long-term. Remember, the Whole30 is a big habit change! It's okay to *not* change everything at once. If joining a CSA, shopping at the farmers market, or making your own bone broth feels intimidating, don't stress about that now! There's plenty of time to expand your healthy dietary habits. For now, your only job is to stick to the Whole30 rules 100%, so let that be enough.

EXTRA CREDIT: Expand your "elevator speech," including two or three personal reasons you started the Whole30, and two or three benefits you've already seen. Then, practice it a few times, ideally out loud or in front of a supportive friend.

At this point in your Whole30 journey, you're probably still focusing on the minutiae: what's happening in your body, how you're feeling, and what you're eating. That's a great place to be right now! Remember, the more detailed your journal entries, the more you'll be able to compare from day to day, and see how far you've come when you need a little extra motivation.

What went well today: ....

....

....

....

....

What could have gone better: ....

....

....

....

What I'll do tomorrow: ....

....

....

....

....

Today's Extra Credit:...

....

....

....

....

....

....

9

Today's NSVs

Energy

The Worst   The Best!

1   2   3   4   5   6   7   8   9   10

NOTES: ....

....

Sleep Quality

The Worst   The Best!

1   2   3   4   5   6   7   8   9   10

NOTES: ....

....

Cravings

The Worst   The Best!

1   2   3   4   5   6   7   8   9   10

NOTES: ....

....

FILL IN YOUR OWN

NSV #1: ....

....

....

NSV #2: ....

....

....

NSV #3: ....

....

....

WHAT I ATE

Favorite!

☐ Meal 1: ....
....
....

☐ Meal 2: ....
....
....

☐ Meal 3: ....
....
....

Extra meal/snack: ....
....
....

Day 9 Reflections

....
....
....
....
....
....
....

9

☐ **I did it! Whole30 Day 9 is in the bag.**

FACT: You are most likely to quit your Whole30 on Days 10 or 11. The newness of the program has worn off. You've experienced lots of the negatives but have yet to see the "magic." You've let your guard down a bit, so thoughts of "just a taste" come creeping in. And while you're *trying* to have a good attitude, you are hyper-aware of all the foods you're choosing not to eat right now. This is hard! Will the results really be as good as "they" say? You are cranky. You are impatient. And the Whole30 is just some stupid challenge anyway.

Deep breath. Your brain is throwing a tantrum because it senses that this time, you're *serious* about making changes, and quick-and-easy rewards will no longer be a regular occurrence. So buckle up, ask for more support, work hard to avoid temptation, and recommit to the process. You know this is way more than a "stupid challenge," and you aren't going give up on yourself.

Melissa's Motivation

This is where you really start to experience the psychological power of your food choices and habits. You've put in a lot of effort to get this far. Your brain demands a reward (you *deserve* it!), but less-healthy food has always been your go-to prize.

You DO deserve a reward, but think about the "treats" you'd normally consume and what need you're expecting them to fulfill. Are you seeing progress and want to celebrate? Are you discouraged and looking for something to cheer you up? Are you anxious about finishing all 30 days, and it's easier to self-sabotage than fail? Remind yourself that food cannot fill that void for you. When has a cupcake ever made you feel accomplished, comforted, or confident? It's time to find another way to meet that need, because you deserve more than the craving-overconsumption-guilt-stress cycle you've been stuck in.

FAQ

THIS IS MY SECOND WHOLE30, AND IT'S HARDER THAN THE FIRST! WHAT GIVES? About 1 in 4 Whole30ers find the first round easier than subsequent rounds. You'd think it'd be the opposite—that once you had the hang of it, future rounds would be a breeze. Here are a few reasons you may struggle:

➤ **YOU KNOW WHAT'S COMING.** It's easier to do something hard without knowing how hard it's going to be. This time, you know the tough parts are ahead, and it's harder to hang in until the magic shows up.

➤ **NO MORE LOW-HANGING FRUIT.** Your first Whole30 was a big change, and you saw equally big transformations. You may not see as dramatic results this time, though, which makes it harder to maintain motivation.

➤ **LACK OF PLANNING.** You thought, "I've done this before… I can wing it." But there is no winging the Whole30, and lack of meal prep, emergency food, and if/then plans have you scrambling so hard, you're thinking of bailing.

Your Round 2 (or 3, or 6) strategy? Plan, prepare, (re)create a support system, keep tracking your NSVs, and finish this program *just* as strong as with your first.

> **COMMUNITY INSPIRATION**
>
> "I have been offered Girl Scout cookies, pastries, and chips at work and it's not even 10 a.m. Refusing is hard, but it's so empowering! I'm just gonna keep refilling my Thermos with coffee and tea while politely thanking my co-workers for their offers. I want that Tiger Blood!" —*Lizabeth M., New York*

10

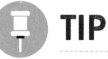

TIP

During the Hardest Days, it's even more important to lean on your support community, in person and online. They can provide extra motivation, like "What do you mean, you're not seeing changes? Your skin looks amazing!" They can offer advice, like, "Sounds like you're not eating enough—what about a post-workout meal?" Or, they can kick you in the booty: "You have birthed a baby and run a marathon. You're not caving because you haven't had *cheese* in ten days." You can even throw out an "SOS" on Whole30 social media; you'll have ten people tossing you a life vest in minutes. There's no shame in asking for help—that's why we're here! Reaching out means you reinforce your commitment, get some much-needed connection, and secure some all-important accountability.

HACK

When it comes to forming habits, expert Gretchen Rubin says treating yourself along the way can bring you more self-control, while depriving yourself of treats can make you feel burned out, deprived, and resentful. (Sound familiar?) You may be so used to rewarding yourself with food that any other form of "treat" hasn't crossed your mind! To best reinforce the habits you are building on the Whole30, give yourself health-minded treats that don't involve food. Try a new kitchen gadget, a yoga mat, a cookbook, or a "date night" at the movie theater (BYO meat sticks). Don't be stingy! Even tiny rewards, like an inspirational coffee mug, can go a long way toward propping up your healthy habits and making you feel gratified.

EXTRA CREDIT: Treat yo'self—even if today wasn't your best day, even if you feel like you're still struggling, even if you "still have a long way to go." You are changing your life one day at a time, and *that* deserves to be rewarded!

If today is feeling extra-tough, counteract that by being extra-generous in today's reflections. Go big in "what went well," and make a robust plan for taking good care of yourself in what you'll do tomorrow. Knock off any and all NSVs you see, no matter how small, and high-five yourself for hitting the one-third point in your Whole30!

What went well today: ....

....

....

....

....

What could have gone better: ....

....

....

....

....

What I'll do tomorrow: ....

....

....

....

....

Today's Extra Credit:..

....

....

....

....

....

....

10

Today's NSVs

Energy
The Worst   The Best!

1   2   3   4   5   6   7   8   9   10

NOTES: ....
....

Sleep Quality
The Worst   The Best!

1   2   3   4   5   6   7   8   9   10

NOTES: ....
....

Cravings
The Worst   The Best!

1   2   3   4   5   6   7   8   9   10

NOTES: ....
....

FILL IN YOUR OWN

NSV #1: ....
....
....

NSV #2: ....
....
....

NSV #3: ....
....
....

WHAT I ATE

Favorite!

☐ Meal 1: ....
....
....
....

☐ Meal 2: ....
....
....

☐ Meal 3: ....
....
....

Extra meal/snack: ....
....
....

Day 10 Reflections

....
....
....
....
....
....

☐ **I did it! Whole30 Day 10 is in the bag.**

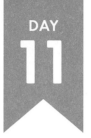

ON DAY 11, you *finally* reach the peak of the roller coaster. You're not over the hump just yet, but from your vantage point, you can see the whole Food Freedom amusement park and feel the anticipation in the air. Your energy is better (if inconsistent), cravings are more manageable, and you're getting the hang of your Whole30 routine. You're confidently turning down off-plan food and using the self-confidence boost as motivation. It's a good day!

If this is you, just enjoy the ride. Eat your food, live your life, use the energy spurts to help you plan and prepare even better for tomorrow, and accept the compliments of others who see that whatever you've been doing is totally working. But if YOUR Day 11 is one of the Hardest Days, coast on through. Don't take on any new Whole30-related challenges, let yourself rest if you need it . . . and make something other than eggs for breakfast, because you're two seconds away from burning out.

Melissa's Motivation

You've been go-go-go on your Whole30; planning meals, prepping food, and doing three days' worth of dishes every night. You're starting to feel better, but you may be experiencing some food fatigue. Like, "If I have to eat another egg muffin/salmon cake/zoodle, I'm gonna lose it." This, in turn, can sap your motivation.

Ready for some tough love? There is no reason to EVER be bored on the Whole30! There are thousands of delicious Whole30 recipes available online or in our cookbooks. Sure, in the beginning, it's easier to eat the same things on repeat. But if you want to turn this into a lifestyle, you're going to *have* to branch out from eggs/bacon/sweet potato. Now that you're more firmly settled in your habits, try some new foods, cooking techniques, spices, or recipes to keep you excited and satisfied.

PLEASE DON'T MAKE ME EAT ANOTHER EGG FOR BREAKFAST. That's not really a question, but we feel you. Let's redefine "Meal 1" and offer some alternatives to eggs on eggs on eggs.

▶ **TRADITIONAL.** Opt for traditional breakfast meats, like sausage, chicken sausage, smoked salmon, or sugar-free ham. Try a sausage, potato, pepper, onion, and kale hash topped with hot sauce, ranch dressing, or pesto.

▶ **BREAKFAST SALAD.** Salads are common for breakfast in Europe, and a light, fresh meal is a great way to start the day. Try salmon cakes or tuna over fresh greens and veggies, with a drizzle of balsamic dressing.

▶ **DINNER FOR BREAKFAST.** You CAN have a burger, steak, or grilled chicken in the morning. Busting out of the breakfast mindset is so liberating, and eating last night's leftovers in the a.m. makes for a hearty, quick, and easy meal before work.

▶ **MIX IT UP.** If you want to keep eggs in the rotation, try them scrambled instead of hard-boiled, top one of the above ideas with an over-easy egg, or make a frittata or egg "muffin," varying the ingredients (meat, veggies, herbs, spices, and sauces) to keep things interesting.

COMMUNITY INSPIRATION

"Last night when I was eating my zoodles, meatballs, and marinara, I thought 'I could eat like this forever.' I am beginning to feel better. My mood is super-fly. A few people have commented that I seem more like myself these days. I'm getting better at this every day!" —*Heather L., Tennessee*

TIP

Though you may be tempted, now is NOT the time to get lazy with your Whole30 habits or take a break from working on your relationship with food. If you've been struggling, you may be tempted to "relax" and indulge with some old, comforting habits. Eating an RxBar as a mid-afternoon pick-me-up and a banana with almond butter for an after-dinner treat may be technically compliant, but that's just feeding your Sugar Dragon and reinforcing the cycle of "craving/emotion/need to comfort --> reward" that you're trying so desperately to break. This part of your Whole30 journey might feel like A LOT. You may be tempted to soften your commitment just a little—after all, you're working hard, and you'd technically still be following the rules. But please, resist. If you just hang in another day or two, digging deep and working hard, you'll be on the downward slope, and *so happy* you didn't wake that snoozing Dragon.

HACK

Habit research shows that one thing that keeps you motivated in a new behavior is accountability—regularly sharing your progress and results with someone else. So why not combine some accountability with restoring excitement to your Whole30 food? Find a health-minded buddy, double your usual prep, then swap compliant meals, dressings, sauces, or side dishes a few times a week. (They don't have to be on the program, but bonus if they are!) Knowing you're going to connect with a friend about your Whole30 will keep you invested, *and* you get some tasty new foods to keep you happy—win/win!

EXTRA CREDIT: Browse through our cookbooks, Real Plans (w30.co/w30realplans), or @whole30recipes on Instagram, and pick a few new recipes to try this week. Even better, if the recipe calls for a kitchen gadget you don't have . . . treat yo'self!

If your journal entries are more upbeat and your NSV section is full, that's a great indicator of things to come. But don't worry if you have yet to see some of the benefits we've talked about. Focus on the things that *are* changing, be patient, and remember the mental and emotional victories you've seen are just as important as the physical.

What went well today: ....

....

....

....

....

What could have gone better: ....

....

....

....

....

What I'll do tomorrow: ....

....

....

....

....

Today's Extra Credit:..

....

....

....

....

....

....

Today's NSVs

Energy

The Worst   The Best!

1 2 3 4 5 6 7 8 9 10

NOTES: ....

Sleep Quality

The Worst   The Best!

1 2 3 4 5 6 7 8 9 10

NOTES: ....

Cravings

The Worst   The Best!

1 2 3 4 5 6 7 8 9 10

NOTES: ....

FILL IN YOUR OWN

NSV #1: ....

....

NSV #2: ....

....

NSV #3: ....

....

WHAT I ATE

Favorite!

☐ Meal 1:...
....
....

☐ Meal 2:...
....
....

☐ Meal 3:...
....
....

Extra meal/snack:...
....
....

Day 11 Reflections

☐ **I did it! Whole30 Day 11 is in the bag.**

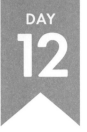

DAY
12

IT'S DAY 12 and you're feeling the downhill momentum. You wake up strangely happy, cautiously optimistic, and feeling pretty darn good. Your Tiger Blood hasn't fully kicked in yet, you may still have some cravings, and the dishes just won't end. BUT, you're tossing your Whole30 lunches together effortlessly; someone offered you donuts at work and you didn't think twice before saying, "No, thanks," and that orange you just ate ... is this what an orange is *supposed* to taste like? It's so pure and sweet ... WHAT IS HAPPENING TO YOU?

Whole30 is happening! Your taste buds are changing, your blood sugar is better regulated, your hormones are doing their job, and your immune system is calming down. Everything is starting to work the way nature intended, so your body is sending you all the right signals. It's not ALL sunshine, rainbows, and ponies from here on out, but if this is you today, throw your hands in the air and enjoy the ride.

Melissa's Motivation

Your good feelings today are also the result of a boost in self-efficacy —your belief in your own ability to succeed. In order to complete all 30 days of your Whole30 totally by the book, you first need to BELIEVE that you can. You may have felt like this in the beginning; on Day 1, your reflections were probably full of self-affirmations, encouragement, and positive thinking. But look back over subsequent days. Were you expressing doubt, anxiety, or fear about the program or your capacity to see your commitment through? (If so, that's totally normal!)

Today, you're feeling better, but more important, you've got 12 days of Whole30 behind you, boosting your belief that you can (and will) finish strong and successfully change your life. Embrace it, and be proud of yourself. I always knew you could do it ... and now you do too.

FAQ ◀

CAN MY TASTE BUDS REALLY BE CHANGING THIS FAST?
The short answer is yes they can, now that you're no longer bombarding them with so much sugar, salt, and fat.

➤ Supernormally stimulating foods are created by scientists to be sweeter, saltier, and fattier than anything you'd find in nature. We call this stuff "food with no brakes" because they're designed to hook our brains with huge hits of pleasure and reward, promoting overconsumption and cravings for more. (Once you start eating them, you just can't stop!) They also overload your taste buds. When you're used to SO much sugar, salt, and fat in a strawberry-frosted donut or a deep-fried onion bloom, you're likely to find fresh strawberries or sautéed onions kind of boring.

➤ Taking a break from supernormally stimulating foods during your Whole30 allows your taste buds to reset—no more overload! Soon, you'll notice more flavor in whole foods, more sweetness in fruit, and that a little bit of salt goes a long way in meals. This reinforces your new, healthy habits, and may lead you to *prefer* the natural sweetness of a strawberry to the artificial, sickly-sweet flavors of your formerly-beloved donut—making it easier to say no when offered. In fact, post-Whole30, you may find your old favorite (processed) treats aren't so delicious anymore ... sorry not sorry.

> COMMUNITY INSPIRATION
>
> "Sat at brunch across from a cheeseburger, French fries, and a root beer. It looked good, but I felt *completely* satiated and happy with my yellowfin tuna salad. My cravings are like, 'Meh,' whereas they used to be 'GIMMMMMMEEEE THAT FOOD!'"
> —*Debbie N., New Jersey*

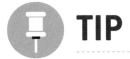

TIP

You can increase your self-efficacy by diving even deeper into the new habits you're building on the Whole30. This will help you reinforce your growth mindset and take small steps toward an overall healthier lifestyle. Pick up a book from a health-minded chef, a manual on home gardening, or the biography of an inspirational health advocate. The next time you want to window-shop, browse a cooking, specialty food, outdoor, or sporting goods store. Actively connect with Whole30 graduates (in person or online), surrounding yourself with healthy role models, asking for advice, and offering your own support where you can. The more invested you become, the more Whole30 self-efficacy you'll build.

HACK

One trick straight out of habit research is to reframe *challenges* as *opportunities* to strengthen your new healthy habits. Being invited to your monthly book club may seem stressful at first; all those off-plan foods and social pressure to enjoy the wine they always serve could make you anxious. But you can boost your self-efficacy by reframing this into an exciting opportunity. What can you bring that will keep you happily munching *and* impress your fellow book club members? How fancy can you make a pitcher of mocktails (and how happy will you be when you wake up clear-headed tomorrow)? Learning to shift your perspective is a handy skill in every area of life, but practicing it here will reinforce your commitment to the program and make you feel even more like a Whole30 rock star.

EXTRA CREDIT: Think of one challenge you're facing this week and turn it into an opportunity. Write down the situation, reframe the obstacles into fun or exciting projects, and create a few if/then plans around how you'll handle the unexpected.

As you reflect on today, give yourself extra-extra credit for all of the good decisions you've made, benefits you're seeing, and challenges you turned into opportunities. The daily practice of journaling your Whole30 is reinforcing your new, healthy habits; reminding you that your commitment to the Whole30 is solid, and boosting your self-efficacy even more.

12

What went well today: ....

....

....

....

What could have gone better: ....

....

....

....

What I'll do tomorrow: ....

....

....

....

Today's Extra Credit: ....

....

....

....

....

....

Today's NSVs

Energy

The Worst   The Best!

1   2   3   4   5   6   7   8   9   10

NOTES: ....

....

Sleep Quality

The Worst   The Best!

1   2   3   4   5   6   7   8   9   10

NOTES: ....

....

Cravings

The Worst   The Best!

1   2   3   4   5   6   7   8   9   10

NOTES: ....

....

FILL IN YOUR OWN

NSV #1: ....

....

....

NSV #2: ....

....

....

NSV #3: ....

....

....

WHAT I ATE

Favorite!

☐ Meal 1: ....

....

....

☐ Meal 2: ....

....

....

☐ Meal 3: ....

....

....

Extra meal/snack: ....

....

Day 12 Reflections

....

....

....

....

....

....

☐ **I did it! Whole30 Day 12 is in the bag.**

IT'S DAY 13—generally a mixed bag. Many of you are starting to feel the magic; sleeping better, energy more consistent, and cravings mostly under control. But lots of you are tired ... either *still* tired, or *back to* tired. You were feeling good, and now you're not as energetic, or your energy fades as the day goes on. This is really common and often means you're not eating enough dietary fat to flip that switch, or enough carbs to fuel your activity levels.

It's common to undereat on the Whole30, especially if you're a little fat-phobic or have weight loss in the back of your mind. But not eating enough leads to more cravings, disrupted sleep, and low energy, all of which can undermine your confidence in the program. Bookmark this entry in case your "I was feeling great, but now I'm tired" shows up later in the program, and use the tips here to get you back on the Tiger Blood track.

Melissa's Motivation

If you've been stuck in a weight-loss mentality (deprivation, restriction, measuring every bite of food), it may feel like you're overeating on the Whole30. Add to that some common-but-temporary side effects like bloating or constipation and you may be tempted to go back to tracking, logging, and micromanaging your meals. Please, don't do this.

Since the Whole30 *isn't* a quick-fix weight loss plan, it may take longer to see the benefits ... and you won't find most of them on the scale. But magical things happen when you start eating real, nutrient-dense, satiating food. It may *feel* like you're eating a lot, but during this process, your body learns to burn fat as fuel, reconnects you with "hungry" and "full" signals, and ditches the sugar cravings. Plus, you hated counting calories, and it never worked for you long-term anyway ... so give our calculator-free process a fair shot!

FAQ

I HAVE AN ACTIVE JOB, WORK LONG DAYS, AM PREGNANT OR NURSING, OR EXERCISE A LOT. ARE THREE MEALS ENOUGH? Probably not. Remember, three meals a day is just a general recommendation! If your context requires more meals or snacks, please do.

13

➤ **ADD A PRE-WORKOUT SNACK AND POST-WORKOUT MEAL.** A pre-workout snack (a little protein, a little fat) like two hard-boiled eggs or an Epic bar can help prepare you for hard work, while a post-workout meal (protein-rich, with healthy carbs) can help you recover from activity. See our meal template (page 6) for details.

➤ **EAT FOUR (OR FIVE) MEALS.** If you have a lot of muscle, work very long days, or are night-nursing, you may need an extra meal (or two) in there. Just try to leave at least 3–4 hours between meals to let your hormones do their job.

➤ **SNACK, IF THAT'S NEEDED.** Many pregnant moms *can't* eat big meals once their baby starts growing, and if you're nursing around the clock, food is "catch it when you can." Feel free to add mini-meals into your day; just don't graze like an antelope ... unless grazing is all you can do in that first trimester! If that's the case, just stick to Whole30 ingredients —food aversions and morning sickness generally do pass.

> **COMMUNITY INSPIRATION**
>
> "After the initial hump, things are a lot better. I have energy for things I usually have no energy to do, like yoga and walks. This is a big deal. Often I have a feeling of intense can't-get-out-of-bed-exhaustion. To have a little more pep in my step feels invaluable." —*Gina E., soletshangout.com*

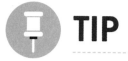

TIP

While the Whole30 recommends filling your plate with vegetables (especially nutrient-dense greens), if you play a high-energy sport like soccer, do mid-distance endurance training (like half-marathons), or perform high-intensity workouts like CrossFit, poor performance might be due to a lack of carbs. While broccoli and kale are nutrient-dense, they're not very *energy*-dense, and these activities demand carbohydrates for optimal fueling. Start adding a fist-sized serving of potatoes, winter squash, beets, and/or fruit to every meal, and be generous post-workout. If lack of carbohydrates was the issue, you'll start feeling better fast. (And feel free to play around with quantity here—you may find a hearty serving of potatoes post-workout feels awesome, but that much at lunchtime leaves you sleepy.)

HACK

The brain has a habit of thinking if SOME is good, MORE is better. Sometimes this is true; if some Whole30 meal prep is good, a more robust plan and extra just-in-case food usually works out for the better. But when it comes to the Whole30 and weight loss, more restriction is definitely *not* better! We know many of you want to see a change in your waistline, so we've built healthy, sustainable weight loss right into our meal template. But restricting fat, carbs, or calories even further will promote cravings, force your willpower into overdrive, *and* slow your metabolism. Trust the process! More isn't better, BETTER is better . . . and the Whole30 is already proving better than *any* weight loss diet.

EXTRA CREDIT: If needed, plan for more healthy carbs in tomorrow's meals, like a banana with lunch or half a sweet potato post-workout. And review the meal template (page 6) to make sure you're eating enough healthy fats!

Sometimes we get so comfortable moving along in the process that we don't even notice we're veering off-course. If your Whole30 meal plan could use some tweaking, use today's reflections to note some action items. Consider meal sizes, macronutrient proportions, and/or the number of meals you're eating. Spend time here, and you'll get to Tiger Blood all the faster!

What went well today: ....

What could have gone better: ....

What I'll do tomorrow: ....

Today's Extra Credit: ....

Today's NSVs

Energy

The Worst   The Best!

1   2   3   4   5   6   7   8   9   10

NOTES: ....

....

Sleep Quality

The Worst   The Best!

1   2   3   4   5   6   7   8   9   10

NOTES: ....

....

Cravings

The Worst   The Best!

1   2   3   4   5   6   7   8   9   10

NOTES: ....

....

FILL IN YOUR OWN

NSV #1: ....

....

NSV #2: ....

....

NSV #3: ....

....

WHAT I ATE

Favorite!

☐ Meal 1: ....
....
....

☐ Meal 2: ....
....
....

☐ Meal 3: ....
....
....

Extra meal/snack: ....
....
....

Day 13 Reflections

....
....
....
....
....
....
....

☐ **I did it! Whole30 Day 13 is in the bag.**

DAY 14—TWO WEEKS! You're sleeping better, your skin is clearer, you're more self-confident, you no longer need a nap at 2 p.m., your pants have extra room, temptations are easier to decline, and/or managing your meal planning and emergency food feels, dare we say it . . . nearly effortless. Is *this* the Tiger Blood of which we speak? On the flip side, food boredom may be setting in, you're still feeling stressed when socializing, and you may be trying to boost your energy by eating more.

For some of you, every morning brings new NSVs. For others, you're definitely noticing improvements, but still struggle with digestion, bloating, energy, or other symptoms. Take heart—the benefits you *are* seeing are a clear sign that you are moving in the right direction, and (time for some tough love) . . . there's a reason it's not called the "Whole14."

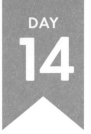 ## Melissa's Motivation

If your Whole30 weather forecast is more "partly sunny" than full sun right now, it's time for a little reframing. You probably went into the Whole30 with some expectations, and maybe they're not all being met just yet. If you're feeling overwhelmed or discouraged, even if it's just in one or two areas, it's time to lose the expectations—because they might be the very thing holding you back!

Every Whole30 is a brand-new experience, and you can't possibly predict what it's going to look like, even if this is your fifth rodeo. So ask yourself . . . if you lost your original expectations, could you be happy with where you are today and the progress you've already made? Spoiler: The answer is almost assuredly yes, so you should do that immediately. Take each day as it comes. Be on the lookout for NSVs. Don't expect anything—but let yourself be pleasantly surprised and proud of yourself as each new day brings something good.

FAQ

SERIOUSLY, CAN WE TALK ABOUT THE DISHES? Okay, sure. All that meal prep, chopping, and cooking can make your dishwasher work overtime—especially if *you're* the dishwasher. Here are some tips for keeping your kitchen neat and clean.

→ **MISE EN PLACE.** Prep all your ingredients before you start cooking, and add ingredients and/or spices that go into the pan at the same time to the same prep bowl. This will give you time to clean as you go.

→ **BUY A BIGGER CUTTING BOARD.** Use one big cutting board for *all* your veggies instead of a few small ones. (Always use a separate one for raw meat.) Bonus: Epicurean brand composite wood boards are quick-dry, so if you want to rinse mid-prep, they're ready to go in a flash!

→ **USE THE SAME PAN.** If you're frying up bacon *and* cooking eggs *and* wilting spinach, cook the bacon first, then use the bacon grease and the hot pan to whip those eggs into shape, then toss the spinach in for a hot minute once the eggs come out.

→ **CLEAN AS YOU GO.** Seriously, you should do this. If you throw onions in the pan and they need two minutes to soften, that's time to wash two dishes or clean the counter scraps. And because you've mise-en-place'd, you don't have anything else to do while they cook!

14

COMMUNITY INSPIRATION

"Today I realized that I've cared more about what I weigh than the true health of my body. I understand now that if this doesn't change, I will *never* lose all the weight that I need to. This is my goal for these 30 days: changing my mindset and changing my life."   *—Sara K., Colorado*

TIP

A few inexpensive kitchen tools can make your Whole30 meal prep so much faster. Try a garlic press instead of manually mincing; a citrus juicer instead of laboriously trying to get the last few drops out by hand; a microplane instead of peeling and chopping your zest; a small "chopper" for salsa, gazpacho, or hash; a variety of small storage containers with lids to save leftover spice mixtures and dressings; half a dozen small bowls for mise-en-place; and buy a second set of measuring cups and spoons, because the tablespoon is *always* in the dishwasher. Oh, and paper plates for *really* busy days, insert praise hands emoji.

HACK

A University of California study measuring stress hormone levels in 30 couples found that people who describe their home environment as "chaotic" or "messy" had higher levels of cortisol (a hormone which helps regulate your body's response to stress) when measured at various points throughout the day. Note: chronically high levels of cortisol wreak havoc in the body, promoting sleeplessness, inflammation, and weight gain, so keeping stress levels down is important! Also interesting: This was more noticeable in women than men. One thing you can take from this is that a tidy kitchen could be a calmer, more confident, happier Whole30 kitchen. One tip straight from Melissa's own playbook: Never go to bed with dishes in the sink. Ten minutes at night is a small sacrifice to wake up to a spotless, gleaming kitchen! (See Day 28's Hack for more.)

EXTRA CREDIT: Do some online shopping or browse your favorite kitchen store and reward yourself with some new gadgets to make your Whole30 faster and easier.

ALTERNATE EXTRA CREDIT: Do all the dishes and wipe the counters before you go to bed tonight!

Release your expectations in tonight's reflection and simply observe *what is*. Mark your NSVs, and pay extra attention to what went well today. Then, go back and re-read your reflections from last week. You may be surprised at how much progress you've actually made, especially when you review it with fresh eyes. (Feel free to high-five yourself here, too!)

What went well today: ....

....

....

....

....

14

What could have gone better: ....

....

....

....

....

What I'll do tomorrow: ....

....

....

....

....

Today's Extra Credit:..

....

....

....

....

....

....

....

Today's NSVs

Energy

The Worst   The Best!

1   2   3   4   5   6   7   8   9   10

NOTES: ....

....

Sleep Quality

The Worst   The Best!

1   2   3   4   5   6   7   8   9   10

NOTES: ....

....

Cravings

The Worst   The Best!

1   2   3   4   5   6   7   8   9   10

NOTES: ....

....

FILL IN YOUR OWN

NSV #1: ....

....

NSV #2: ....

....

NSV #3: ....

....

WHAT I ATE

Favorite!

☐ Meal 1:...
....
....

☐ Meal 2:...
....
....

☐ Meal 3:...
....
....

Extra meal/snack:...
....
....

14

Day 14 Reflections

....
....
....
....
....
....

☐ **I did it! Whole30 Day 14 is in the bag.**

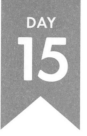

IT'S DAY 15—hey hey, halfway! At this point, you've ~~survived~~ conquered TWO Whole30 weekends, and you're finding it easier to say no to temptations and navigate social situations. Plus, your taste buds are changing—the strawberry, sweet potato, or grapes you just ate was nearly a religious experience, and real food has *never* tasted better. And as your blood sugar is better regulated, you're no longer getting "I'm starving, need sugar" or "I'm tired, need sugar" signals, all of which makes it easier to pass on the birthday cake in the break room or dessert at family dinner.

Not to mention you're fast approaching the Tiger Blood stage—in fact, some of you are *already* feeling it! So congratulate yourself for making it 50% of the way through your Whole30, and get excited, because there's a lot of sunshine, rainbows, and puppies (i.e., *good stuff*) headed your way.

Melissa's Motivation

You're at the halfway mark—and the next two weeks are going to FLY BY. Prediction: At some point, someone will ask you what day you're on, and you'll say, "You know, I don't actually remember." This is winning! You already feel like a Whole30-ish diet (including the foods and drinks you decide are worth it after your reintroduction) could be your forever lifestyle.

However, it's possible that to get this far, you've turned yourself into a Whole30 hermit. Declining social invitations can be a good strategy in the beginning, especially if the event isn't special and you know you'll struggle with temptation. But at this point in your Whole30, you need to start practicing being confident in your health-minded choices in *any* setting—including business lunches, bridal showers, family dinners, or happy hours. It's time . . . and I promise, you're ready. (Or you will be, after today's entries!)

FAQ ◀━━━━━

WHAT ARE YOUR BEST TIPS FOR SOCIAL SITUATIONS?
There are three chapters in *Food Freedom Forever* all about friends, family, and food, but here are the bullet points.

━━━━▶ **PLAN AND PREP.** Eat before you go; research the menu ahead of time; bring your own dressing, coconut aminos, compliant side dish, or emergency food; and create if/then plans for unexpected situations (IF I'm offered a beer, THEN I'll say, "Thanks, but I'm sticking to water tonight," and change the subject).

━━━━▶ **BE CONFIDENT.** Be *totally* confident in your restaurant order. "I'll have the burger, no bun, no cheese, and instead of fries, can I have steamed mixed vegetables, please?" The bigger a deal you make out of your dietary choices, the more you'll call attention to them, so place your order like it ain't no thing and return to the conversation.

━━━━▶ **DO SOCIALIZE!** You *can* bond with co-workers at happy hour just as effectively with sparkling water in your glass, and you may even enjoy it more (especially the next morning). Remember that social encounters aren't about the food on your plate; they're about the people you're with, the connections you make, and the memories you create.

COMMUNITY INSPIRATION

"Last night at our local Mexican restaurant, I had a club soda and lime. It wasn't hard because I know that I'm not going to be bloated or have acid reflux in an hour. I'm reminding myself why I *don't want to eat it* instead of telling myself I *can't have it.* And it's working!"   —Lisa J., Oregon

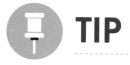

TIP

The most powerful three words in your Whole30 socialization arsenal: a very pleasant "No, thank you." Your Whole30 will get a lot more social once you get comfortable with the idea that these three words are a complete sentence all by themselves. The key is to practice! Don't be defensive, or feel the need to justify or explain. Your choices are your choices, so stand by them confidently! Practice saying, "No, thank you" or "I'm good, thanks" or "Not tonight, thanks," and then move on by changing the subject, asking a question, or taking a pointed sip of your sparkling water. The more matter-of-fact and confident you are here, the less you'll have to contend with a second offering—or worse, peer pressure to have "just one." (But if that does happen, a second "Again, no, but thanks" with direct eye contact and a smile will almost assuredly do the trick.)

HACK

Need more reasons to get out there and be social? Studies have shown that having a support network contributes significantly to your psychological well-being. Connecting with "your people" can bring you a sense of belonging, an increased sense of self-worth, and a feeling of security. It's also been shown to modulate stress and improves your coping ability when times get tough—which can come in handy during a Whole30! Don't cut yourself off from the social support you deserve during your program. Take advantage of all of the benefits of connecting with good people while building self-confidence around food and temptation.

EXTRA CREDIT: Be more social this week—plan a golf outing, host a casual dinner with friends, or RSVP to your niece's birthday party. Make a plan, create some if/then scenarios in case you need them . . . then get out there and enjoy yourself!

Use today's reflections to help you plan for social situations, but also to remind yourself of all of the benefits you're already seeing during your Whole30. The more confident you are that this program is working for you (and the more effectively you can articulate exactly *how* it's working for you), the better you'll be able to connect with those who want to support you.

What went well today: ---

What could have gone better: ---

15

What I'll do tomorrow: --

Today's Extra Credit:---

Today's NSVs

Energy

The Worst   The Best!

1   2   3   4   5   6   7   8   9   10

NOTES: ....

....

Sleep Quality

The Worst   The Best!

1   2   3   4   5   6   7   8   9   10

NOTES: ....

....

Cravings

The Worst   The Best!

1   2   3   4   5   6   7   8   9   10

NOTES: ....

....

FILL IN YOUR OWN

NSV #1: ....

....

....

NSV #2: ....

....

....

NSV #3: ....

....

....

WHAT I ATE

Favorite!

☐ Meal 1:...
....
....

☐ Meal 2:...
....
....

☐ Meal 3:...
....
....

Extra meal/snack:...
....
....

15

Day 15 Reflections

....
....
....
....
....
....
....

☐ **I did it! Whole30 Day 15 is in the bag.**

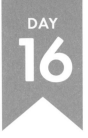

DAY

16

IT'S DAY 16 . . . what were you doing last night? Did you chow down on tacos, tortilla chips, and cold cervezas? Did you eat half a cheesecake with your hands? Wait, you don't even like cheesecake? Well *that* hardly matters when it comes to your Whole30 food dreams!

Nearly all Whole30ers report at least one dream where you're going to town on non-compliant food. Sometimes, it's a food you'd never eat in real life. Often, you wake up feeling guilty, embarrassed, or disappointed in yourself. This is all totally normal! You've been uniquely preoccupied with food for the last 15 days, and your brain does weird things when you tell it "No." Chalk it up to a side effect of changing your emotional relationship with food, shake it off by reminding yourself that it was JUST A DREAM . . . and next time you find yourself pretend-eating, try to enjoy it, because Whole30 rules don't apply in dreams!

Melissa's Motivation

By now, you've had more than a few opportunities to say "No, thank you" in the face of treats, drinks, or other off-plan foods, and at least a few times, it's felt nearly effortless or automatic. This is a *huge* NSV that you may be overlooking—so let me shine a light for you.

If you've been focusing on your expectations ("I thought I'd have zero cravings by now") or your struggles ("I almost gave in last night"), you may be missing the slow-but-steady way your habits and relationship with food are changing. You love how it feels to feed yourself well. You're developing comforting practices that don't involve opening the pantry. Your self-efficacy is high. You're starting to *feel* like a healthy person with healthy habits. And if even once you casually take a pass on something you used to automatically accept (and overconsume), I'd mark that as a MAJOR win—and you should too!

FAQ ◀━━━━━━

SHOULD I BE REWARDING MYSELF DURING MY WHOLE30 JOURNEY? YES . . . but not how you used to! You're trying to break the emotional association between "food" and "self-love" here, so letting yourself finally have that Coconut Cacao RxBar you've been craving is seriously missing the point. Instead, Gretchen Rubin (author of the habit book *Better Than Before*) suggests you choose a reward that takes you deeper into the habit you're trying to establish. Here are two great areas to explore, but any "treat" that solidifies your commitment to healthy habits would work.

━━━▶ GET COOKING. You're spending more time in the kitchen, preparing meals by hand and reaping/eating the benefits of your hard work. Seems like the perfect opportunity to reward yourself with a new kitchen gadget, pretty dinnerware, a high-end chef's knife, a cast-iron pan, a set of Primal Palate spice blends, or a local cooking or knife-skills class.

━━━▶ GET MOVING. While there is no exercise component to the Whole30, many people report that having more energy makes them want to be more active, so choose a reward that encourages you to get out there. Motivate yourself with new sneakers or yoga tights, a membership at TMACfitness.com or your local fitness studio, a few sessions with a personal trainer, a new backpack for hiking, or a pair of wireless headphones.

16

COMMUNITY INSPIRATION

"I dreamed I woke up, went to the kitchen, and ate ONE white chocolate–covered pretzel. When I woke up, I was convinced it was real and wanted to cry. Once I realized it wasn't, I promptly threw away the *real* white chocolate–covered pretzels (in my pantry). Can't haunt me now!"   —Molly J.

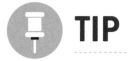

TIP

Don't let food dreams throw you—you aren't doing anything wrong, and they're not a "bad sign." People on crash diets often dream about food because they're deprived of calories and micronutrition, which can lead to unhealthy obsessions while awake *and* asleep—but this isn't your scenario. You're eating real, nutritious food, and not restricting calories. The dreams are likely a representation of how committed you are to the process . . . and how much you've occasionally missed your bread, wine, or cheese. You don't have to feel guilty about what you do in dreams. In fact, if you can recognize you're dreaming, you might as well enjoy it! (Though it may feel like it, Melissa *cannot* see inside your dreams—they're a Whole30-free zone.)

HACK

Author Charles Duhigg (*The Power of Habit*) says that every habit has three parts: the cue, the routine, and the reward. Sometimes, you can hack a bad habit by changing the cue; if morning break room treats are tempting, save your visit until after lunch. But sometimes, the cue just IS . . . it's always going to be 3 p.m., or you're always going to come home from work. If you can't change it, try to find a different routine (not involving food) to satisfy the same reward. That mid-afternoon boost you're looking for could come from chatting with a co-worker or getting outside for a few minutes, and your new post-work wind-down could involve some fun music or taking your dog for a walk. Same cue, satisfying reward . . . but a much healthier routine.

EXTRA CREDIT: Map out some exciting rewards that can keep you motivated and engaged in your new habits and growth mind-set. Make a list of ways to treat yourself along the way, then commit to doing nice things for yourself throughout the process. You deserve it!

Use this space to reflect on your Whole30 habits, and how your emotional relationship with food has been changing. Confidently mark down even small progress as measurable progress. Then, identify a few Whole30 areas of focus on which you'd like to expand, because we'll have plenty of guidance for taking your Whole30 practice even deeper in the coming days.

What went well today: ....

What could have gone better: ....

16

What I'll do tomorrow: ....

Today's Extra Credit: ....

Today's NSVs

Energy

The Worst   The Best!

1   2   3   4   5   6   7   8   9   10

NOTES: ....

....

Sleep Quality

The Worst   The Best!

1   2   3   4   5   6   7   8   9   10

NOTES: ....

....

Cravings

The Worst   The Best!

1   2   3   4   5   6   7   8   9   10

NOTES: ....

....

FILL IN YOUR OWN

NSV #1: ....

....

....

NSV #2: ....

....

....

NSV #3: ....

....

....

WHAT I ATE

Favorite!

☐ Meal 1:..

....

....

☐ Meal 2:..

....

....

☐ Meal 3:..

....

....

Extra meal/snack:..

....

....

Day 16 Reflections

....
....
....
....
....
....

☐ **I did it! Whole30 Day 16 is in the bag.**

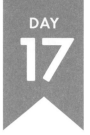

IT'S DAY 17, and for most Whole30ers, that spells TIGER BLOOD! The phrase originated with Charlie Sheen, but we adopted it to describe the consistent energy, happy mood, rockin' self-confidence, and NSVs you're feeling at this point in your Whole30 journey. Of course, your mileage may vary, and your health history, past dietary habits, and lifestyle factors (like stress) all play a role. Some people wake up one day and feel like a switch has been flipped—Energizer Bunny mode ON! Others observe a slow, gradual improvement in markers like energy or cravings ... and still others need another week or two of adaptation before the magic kicks in. So don't be disheartened if your tiger is still napping in the jungle. You still have two weeks left, and your time *will* come.

Melissa's Motivation

If you're part of a Whole30 support community or follow other people's Whole30 journeys online, you're probably taking a ton of motivation, inspiration, encouragement, and resources from these networks. But there is one word of caution in connecting with others during the program: Comparison is the thief of Whole30 joy. Just because your forum friend (who started on the same day) has gone down a pant size or this guy in your gym is killing his workouts doesn't mean you'll have the same experience ... or that you're doing anything wrong if you don't!

The Timeline provides a general frame of reference for what most people experience along the way, but it's not a one-size-fits-all—*especially* when it comes to Tiger Blood. There are so many factors that influence your Whole30 progress and your own measures of "success," including your expectations. Stay focused on your own experience, embrace the good things that ARE happening, and be proud of your *own* journey, wherever you are.

FAQ

I'M NOT FEELING TIGER BLOOD YET. ANY TIPS? Sometimes, small tweaks can make a big difference in your Tiger Blood status. Here are two that can help.

EAT MORE (OR EAT DIFFERENT STUFF). If you're pretty active in your job or exercise routine and eating too low-carb or low-fat, you're gonna feel lethargic, and your performance will suffer. Adding more starchy carbs (like potatoes or winter squash) and fruit to each meal, and/or upping your fat intake, can flip things into high gear. Or, if you're overeating dried fruit, fruit-and-nut bars, or fruit smoothies/juices, you may be sabotaging effective fat adaption by giving yourself sugar too often! Lean more on healthy fats and lower-carb veggies for a week and see if that does the trick.

STOP GRAZING/SNACKING. If you're continuing to eat every 2–3 hours or consistently snacking/grazing between meals, you could be putting the brakes on your body learning how to generate steady, even energy. Your hormones need time between meals to do their job and let you tap into body and dietary fat for energy! If this behavior is habitual, create more awareness around the habit. If it's because you're truly hungry between meals, immediately start making each meal bigger, and continue doing that until three (or four, if you're active) meals a day are doing the trick.

17

COMMUNITY INSPIRATION

"I haven't felt a 'Tiger Blood' magical burst of energy. What I DO feel is steady, continuous energy throughout the day. I wake up more easily and earlier, sleep through the night more, and don't run out of energy every afternoon. Everyone's experience is different, but I love mine!" —*Kristen H.*

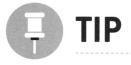

TIP

Life stressors have a profound influence on your health, happiness, *and* Whole30 results. If you're only sleeping five hours a night, over-training, or feel pretty stressed in general, these factors will affect your Tiger Blood. The good news is that an anti-inflammatory diet is a powerful modulator of physical stress, and knowing that one area of your life is under control can alleviate psychological stress too. Change what you can (an earlier bedtime is always a good idea), but otherwise just do your best. Stick to the rules, but don't try to do the "perfect" Whole30, and understand that surviving an incredibly stressful time without breaking down mentally or getting sick may be the best "Tiger Blood" you could hope for.

HACK

Expectations are like a mental shortcut, letting you arrive at a reasonably reliable conclusion with half the effort. Often, expectations are met—but sometimes they do nothing but hold you back, killing your joy, stifling your motivation, and keeping you stuck. You may have more afternoon focus, an easier time waking, and less belly bloat—all amazing results thus far! But if you EXPECTED a dramatic energy surge, blissful sleep, or a drop in pant size by Day X, you may be disappointed with the results you *have* achieved. The key here is to stick to expectations you can control ("I expect to stay committed to this process"), and then stay focused on what you ARE seeing as a result. This will help you find joy in even the smallest improvements.

EXTRA CREDIT: If tweaks are needed to your meal plan, jot down tomorrow's improvements here . . . or, use this space to release your expectations and create a gratitude list of all of the things you are thankful for at this point in your Whole30 journey.

Focus heavily on your NSVs today, being as generous as possible. If you think your meal plan could use some tweaks, note them here, but resist the urge to micromanage. Adding half an apple or one tablespoon of oil isn't going to make or break your Whole30 Tiger Blood. Look for big-picture changes that may help, but if all is well, commit to patience and consistency!

What went well today: ....

....

....

....

What could have gone better: ....

....

....

....

What I'll do tomorrow: ....

....

....

....

Today's Extra Credit: ....

....

....

....

....

....

....

17

Today's NSVs

Energy

The Worst   The Best!

1   2   3   4   5   6   7   8   9   10

NOTES: ....

....

Sleep Quality

The Worst   The Best!

1   2   3   4   5   6   7   8   9   10

NOTES: ....

....

Cravings

The Worst   The Best!

1   2   3   4   5   6   7   8   9   10

NOTES: ....

....

FILL IN YOUR OWN

NSV #1: ....

....

NSV #2: ....

....

NSV #3: ....

....

WHAT I ATE

Favorite!

☐ Meal 1: ....

....

....

☐ Meal 2: ....

....

....

☐ Meal 3: ....

....

....

Extra meal/snack: ....

....

Day 17 Reflections

....

....

....

....

....

....

☐ **I did it! Whole30 Day 17 is in the bag.**

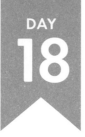

DAY 18

GOOD MORNING, DAY 18! At this point in your Whole30 journey, you may be having GOOD mornings indeed. You're falling asleep faster, sleeping more deeply, and waking up earlier, refreshed and energized. In fact, you've come to realize that sleep is actually the BEST THING EVER.

This is one of the coolest and most underrated Whole30 NSVs. Sleep is where it's at—not enough messes up basically everything, but better sleep can HELP mood, focus, energy, and even weight loss. If you're finding some areas of sleep are better (falling asleep faster) but others are worse (waking more frequently), know this is normal as hormonal rhythms shift. Use these tips to help you maximize your time in bed, and remember there is no shame in a 9 p.m. bedtime game when you're sleeping THIS well.

Melissa's Motivation

In today's overscheduled world, it's a badge of honor to be exhausted. We brag about how busy we are, how little we sleep, and how hard we work. It feels lazy and selfish to go to bed early or practice other forms of basic self-care. Happily, this is NOT the case in Whole30-land, and your relationship with sleep and "busy-ness" is another thing you'll likely improve during your 30 days.

Getting more sleep is a radical act of self-love, leaving you more effective and efficient during your day. Carving out time for yourself makes you happier and healthier—and better able to care for others. As you feel better, you'll want to practice more self-care, which makes you feel even better. OUR cycle rejects the culture of "busy" and reinforces the growth mindset that you are a healthy person with healthy habits. So if you've been feeling guilty for caring for yourself more, STOP. You deserve it, every last bit. And I'm so happy you're loving yourself enough to start giving back to *you*.

FAQ

WHAT ARE YOUR FAVORITE TRICKS FOR GETTING THE BEST NIGHT'S SLEEP? You mean *besides* doing the Whole30? Here are some tips in two major areas from sleep expert Kirk Parsley, MD.

PRE-BED HABITS. The "blue lights" emanating from your smartphone, tablet, or television are especially disruptive at night, suppressing melatonin secretion and messing with your sleep. Your best practice is to have zero screen-time in the hour before bed. (This advice pulls double-duty, as eliminating Facebook/Twitter/email also keeps you from reading something inflammatory or unsettling, which can stress you out and keep you awake.) It's also ideal to finish all exercise sessions at least three hours before bed—*especially* high-intensity activity, which can ramp up cortisol production at a time when it's supposed to be low.

YOUR BEDTIME ENVIRONMENT. Studies show you sleep best in a cool, dark room. Hang blackout curtains, remove or turn off all electronics (anything with a light or glow, including an alarm clock or night light), and if you sleep with your phone in the room, make sure it's on "airplane mode." Turn the heat down; the ideal temp for sleep is between 64 and 68 degrees Fahrenheit. Finally, send yourself off to sleep peacefully using techniques like 4-7-8 breathing or progressive muscle relaxation (see Hack).

18

COMMUNITY INSPIRATION

"Falling asleep has always been a real challenge. I have been on and off of sleep medication for seven years. But on Whole30, WOW. I fell asleep naturally . . . as soon as my head hit the pillow. This was probably the most drastic and exciting change that I experienced on the program."

—*Micaela E.*, Woman's Day

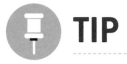

TIP

The Whole30 often helps you sleep better … but you may sleep *worse* first. The protocol will help your body transition back to "insulin sensitivity" (effective blood sugar regulation), but that transition can also cause sleep disruptions, like waking more frequently or earlier than usual. Shifting most of your carbohydrate intake to the last meal of the day might help—so eat plenty of leafy greens, low-carb veggies, and a little fruit at breakfast and lunch; and save the potatoes, winter squash, and bigger servings of fruit for dinner. An all-natural sleep supplement can also make a huge difference. We worked with Dr. Parsley to develop a Whole30 Approved version of his popular Sleep Remedy, which has a reported 85% success rate for improving sleep. (docparsley.com)

HACK

Originally designed to help people with anxiety release tension, progressive muscle relaxation is also an effective practice to help you sleep. (Aside: Melissa has been using this technique for years.) Start at one end of the body—like feet—and contract the muscles hard for a count of five. Then, release all tension and allow them to completely relax. Do this a few times, then move up to your calves. The contraction before relaxation helps your body let go of lingering tension, and teaches your muscles what it feels like to actually relax. Continue working your way up the body until you reach your neck … but there's a good chance you'll fall asleep well before that.

EXTRA CREDIT: Gear up for the best night's sleep of your life by taking some (or all) of the steps outlined here. Unplug electronics, turn down the thermostat, put down your phone, get your Sleep Remedy ready, and compare tonight's sleep to previous days' NSV notations.

In the first two weeks, you were hyper-focused on the technicalities of the program, your food, and meal planning and preparation. Now, you're starting to focus on some of the nuances, and gradually improving some healthy habits tangential to your Whole30 experience. You *could* mark this down as an NSV all on its own today—and you should!

What went well today: ....

....

....

....

....

What could have gone better: ....

....

....

....

What I'll do tomorrow: ....

....

....

....

....

Today's Extra Credit: ....

....

....

....

....

....

....

18

Today's NSVs

Energy

The Worst   The Best!

1   2   3   4   5   6   7   8   9   10

NOTES: ....

....

Sleep Quality

The Worst   The Best!

1   2   3   4   5   6   7   8   9   10

NOTES: ....

....

Cravings

The Worst   The Best!

1   2   3   4   5   6   7   8   9   10

NOTES: ....

....

FILL IN YOUR OWN

NSV #1: ....

....

....

NSV #2: ....

....

....

NSV #3: ....

....

....

WHAT I ATE

Favorite!

☐ Meal 1:...

....

....

☐ Meal 2:...

....

....

☐ Meal 3:...

....

....

Extra meal/snack:...

....

....

Day 18 Reflections

....

....

....

....

....

....

....

18

☐ **I did it! Whole30 Day 18 is in the bag.**

DAY
19

IT'S DAY 19, and you are cruising along. Energy, sleep, focus, and mood have improved. Hunger and cravings are evening out, meal prep is becoming habit, and you're noticing more NSVs every day. But even with all of these benefits, your *waistline* may not be cooperating . . . and that can be a belly-bummer.

Bloating is common on the program, especially early on as your digestive tract starts to heal, the gut bacteria population starts to shift, and your body gets used to eating more vegetables and fat. The Timeline generally points to Days 8–9 as "Why are my pants TIGHTER?" days, and if that's when you experienced it, it's probably disappeared by now. But bloating or other digestive issues *can* persist into the third week. While it could go away on its own, there may be some dietary tweaks you can make to help speed up the adjustment process.

Melissa's Motivation

Don't you wish you could stick a sensor somewhere on your body to show you everything going on inside and how you could fix anything undesirable? It can be really frustrating to take huge, brave steps to change your health, only to feel stuck (or go backwards) in a few areas. If you're still experiencing some not-so-awesome health issues or missing out on some of the key benefits the Whole30 *could* bring, don't be discouraged. You're making HUGE strides, even if your body is taking a little longer to catch up in some areas.

You're asking a lot of all of your body systems right now—heal, calm, regulate, balance—and your body may be slow to respond. We'll help you troubleshoot here, but instead of focusing on the one area that isn't where you want it (yet), remember to be happy with and proud of the positive changes you ARE seeing. This life-changing stuff is hard, but you're doing a great job.

FAQ

WHY AM I STILL GETTING BLOATED? We can't answer that definitively, but there may be some tweaks you can make that will help your body better digest the healthy stuff you're eating.

→ **VEGETABLES AND FRUIT.** Yes, vegetables and fruit are good for you, but this might be a case of too much too soon, or too *raw* too often. Raw vegetables can be harder to digest, especially if you're coming to the Whole30 with a gut condition (IBS, IBD, Crohn's, etc.). And certain "high-FODMAP" vegetables or fruits tend to promote bloating more than others. Your fixes: Try eating most of your vegetables cooked instead of making giant salads. Try breaking up fruit into smaller quantities, like half a serving at a time. Or, visit IBSDiets.org to see list of high-FODMAP produce to avoid. (Tip: Print a copy of the Whole30 Shopping List found at whole30.com/pdf-resources, cross off high-FODMAP veggies and fruit, and eat from the rest for a week to see if that helps.)

→ **DIGESTIVE SUPPORT.** You might just need a little extra help breaking down the protein, fat, or carbohydrates in your Whole30 food. Low-grade inflammation, the aging process, or chronic stress can all impact your body's ability to properly digest. A digestive enzyme and some probiotics could help. See pages 74–77 in *The Whole30* for more details.

COMMUNITY INSPIRATION

"Before Whole30, I had no idea that the way I felt after meals wasn't normal. I can remember nights where I would lie down and "stretch out" my stomach because it hurt after dinner. Now I know what it feels like to be full and satisfied but not bloated or in pain." —*Christina, hungrymeetshealthy.com*

19

🅣 TIP

While fermented foods like kombucha or sauerkraut are all the rage for their gut-health benefits, they may not be helping *your* digestion. Dysbiosis—a disruption in gut bacteria population—and FODMAP intolerance are common in those coming to the Whole30. In these cases, fermented foods can make digestive symptoms worse. In addition, those with histamine sensitivities may find that fermented foods cause headaches, hives, and fatigue. If you've been eating lots of fermented foods and find your digestion isn't awesome, your best bet is to find a functional medicine doctor (see page 406 in *The Whole30*) and do some lab tests. Barring that, try cutting WAY back to small doses (like a tablespoon of sauerkraut a day) and ease back in slowly.

HACK

Sometimes, the simplest solution is the most effective. If certain foods in your Whole30 diet aren't working well for your body, a simple food journal can help you pinpoint the cause. Use the reflection space here or keep a log on your smartphone or laptop, tracking the foods and beverages you consume and the symptoms you experience. If you have a suspicion about any one food, do an elimination inside the Whole30, like "no eggs for three days," and see if symptoms subside. Or go big and eliminate all high-FODMAP foods for a week, slowly adding them back in during the remainder of your Whole30 to help you identify the suspects.

EXTRA CREDIT: If you're still having trouble, bust out *The Whole30* and brush up on Supplements and Troubleshooting. (Also check out Special Populations if you have a gut condition, autoimmune condition, or have had your gallbladder removed.) Or, Google "Whole30 Probiotics 101" and "Whole30 Digestive Enzymes 101" for our articles, courtesy of Dr. Tim Gerstmar.

We spent a lot of time troubleshooting today, but keep the focus of today's reflections positive! If you've been struggling with digestive issues, you now have some great new resources to help you. If you're feeling awesome and everything is clicking, then rack up those NSVs and use today's Extra Credit time to just relax and enjoy your Whole30 benefits.

What went well today: ....

....

....

....

What could have gone better: ....

....

....

....

What I'll do tomorrow: ....

....

....

....

Today's Extra Credit: ....

....

....

....

....

....

19

Today's NSVs

Energy

The Worst   The Best!

1   2   3   4   5   6   7   8   9   10

NOTES: ....

....

Sleep Quality

The Worst   The Best!

1   2   3   4   5   6   7   8   9   10

NOTES: ....

....

Cravings

The Worst   The Best!

1   2   3   4   5   6   7   8   9   10

NOTES: ....

....

FILL IN YOUR OWN

NSV #1: ....

....

....

NSV #2: ....

....

....

NSV #3: ....

....

....

WHAT I ATE

Favorite!

☐ Meal 1: ....

....

....

☐ Meal 2: ....

....

....

☐ Meal 3: ....

....

....

Extra meal/snack: ....

....

....

Day 19 Reflections

....

....

....

....

....

....

....

19

☐ **I did it! Whole30 Day 19 is in the bag.**

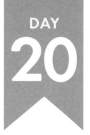

DAY
20

DAY 20 IS A MILE MARKER; just ten days to go—home stretch! It has you thinking, "Now I KNOW I've got this!" (We never had any doubts, but maybe you did.) But while ten days to go can be an exciting prospect, Day 20 is a reminder that you *only have ten days left*. Which might lead to, "I'm not there yet. I'm still snacking/overeating/craving/emotionally eating. I thought I'd be farther along by now. I'm scared I won't figure it out."

This is normal. (We keep saying that, but it bears repeating.) You've never done anything like the Whole30 before—but you've got plenty of experience with *diets*. Diets that don't change your habits or emotional relationship with food, and leave you primed for a major rebound when the program is over. You fear the same pattern here—but remember, this is not that! We've got you covered with the Whole30, reintroduction, and the Food Freedom plan.

Melissa's Motivation

If you're a little freaked out . . . deep breath. These things take time. So you've been 100% compliant for 20 days but still find yourself having cravings, overeating, emotionally eating, or mindlessly snacking? NO BIG DEAL. Of course you don't have it all figured out just yet. Of course you'll struggle along the way. Of course it's scary. Just keep working the program.

Your body is changing. Your tastes are changing. Your brain is changing. YOU are changing. This will not happen overnight, but it *will* happen. And even if it takes you a few years to truly find your food freedom, every day between now and then things will be better, and will continue to get better. Sometimes in big leaps, sometimes by inches, sometimes in the form of two steps backward and a hard-earned three steps forward . . . but progress is progress. Have faith—not just faith in the Whole30, but faith in yourself.

FAQ

HOW CAN I FEEL BETTER PREPARED FOR DAY 31? The Whole30 community says there is one thing that has made them feel so much better (less anxious, more confident, better prepared) for their Whole30 Day 31—reading *Food Freedom Forever* (whole30.com/fooodfreedom) *during* their Whole30. Here's a preview:

→ **LIFE AFTER THE WHOLE30.** *Food Freedom Forever* outlines a plan for "life after the Whole30," helping you use what you learned during your program to create the perfect, sustainable diet for you. It guides you through reintroduction and evaluating the impact of the foods you're bringing back in, but more important, it teaches you how to use that information to make the right decision for you *in the moment*: "Is it worth it? Do I really want it?"

→ **THE FFF 3-PART PLAN.** Perhaps the most comforting part, however, is that FFF trains you to lose the old "diet mentality" (deprive, starve, lose some weight, binge, experience guilt and shame, regain weight, repeat) and start thinking about your food freedom as a life-long cycle. The Food Freedom plan (reset, enjoy your food freedom, acknowledge your healthy habits are starting to slip, repeat) is designed to keep you living your food freedom for longer and longer periods, requiring fewer resets over time . . . while removing guilt, shame, deprivation, or rebounds from the equation.

COMMUNITY INSPIRATION

"It's easy to look at where I am versus where I want to be and the distance between can be discouraging. But this is not a 'diet and done' scenario. This is a 'get to the core of the issues and wrestle and fail and succeed (repeat)' lifestyle shift."

—*Kristen C., Florida*

20

135

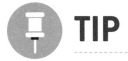

TIP

Think of the Whole30 and your food freedom journey like you think about fitness. You don't do one 30-day boot camp and think, "I'm in shape, I'll never have to do that again!" You know that fitness is a process, requiring dedication and continued effort. You'll have ups and downs, times where it feels effortless and times where you'll slack . . . but as long as you stay committed to the process, you'll stay fit and healthy. The Whole30 is just like that. You'll probably need more than one reset, but doing another Whole30 *isn't* a sign of failure! It's just like signing up for another boot camp—you, recommitting to the process with some added support and structure, until you once again feel solid in your habits.

HACK

The brain LOVES a plan, but this is especially true if you're an "abstainer," someone who thrives in black-and-white rules and doesn't do well with moderation. For you, leaving the comfort of the Whole30 might be extra-scary, which is why having a plan to keep you looking and feeling your best after the Whole30 is over is even more important. The framework outlined in *Food Freedom Forever* will set your mind at ease that once you're out there "riding your own bike" during reintroduction and the days to follow, you'll have a concrete plan designed to keep you firmly entrenched in your new, healthy habits. (And Google "Whole30 Abstainer or Moderator" for an article on how these two groups should approach food freedom.)

EXTRA CREDIT: Pick up, borrow, or download the audio version of *Food Freedom Forever* and start reading or listening . . . tonight! Bonus: Diving into this subject matter will strengthen your growth mind-set, reaffirming that even after your Whole30 is over, you're still a healthy person with healthy habits.

Today we focused on looking ahead, but there are tons of amazing things happening right now—in the present. It's time to jump back into your Day 20 reflections, focusing specifically on what went well today and whether you're noticing any new NSVs (or improvements in current ones) at this point in your journey. Feeling good? Bring on the final ten days!

What went well today: _____

_____

_____

_____

_____

What could have gone better: _____

_____

_____

_____

_____

What I'll do tomorrow: _____

_____

_____

_____

_____

Today's Extra Credit: _____

_____

_____

_____

_____

_____

_____

20

Today's NSVs

Energy

The Worst   The Best!

1   2   3   4   5   6   7   8   9   10

NOTES: ....

....

Sleep Quality

The Worst   The Best!

1   2   3   4   5   6   7   8   9   10

NOTES: ....

....

Cravings

The Worst   The Best!

1   2   3   4   5   6   7   8   9   10

NOTES: ....

....

FILL IN YOUR OWN

NSV #1: ....

....

....

NSV #2: ....

....

....

NSV #3: ....

....

....

WHAT I ATE

Favorite!

☐ Meal 1: ....
....
....

☐ Meal 2: ....
....
....

☐ Meal 3: ....
....
....

Extra meal/snack: ....
....
....

Day 20 Reflections

....
....
....
....
....
....

20

☐ **I did it! Whole30 Day 20 is in the bag.**

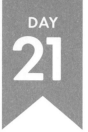

IF DAY 20 HAD YOU NERVOUS that you only had ten more days to figure things out, Day 21 might have you thinking, "NINE more days? I'm so over this." It's common to feel burned out at this stage—you're three weeks into it, but the light at the end of this health and habit tunnel is still just a little too far off to be encouraging. Also, nothing sounds good for breakfast. Nothing. DON'T EVEN THINK ABOUT SHOWING ME ANOTHER EGG.

You're loving the way your body is responding during the program, but the idea of making it to the end sounds like drudgery. Really, though, you're probably just bored. Bored with your food, bored with the routine, bored with the dishes, just . . . bored. So let's use today's tips and hacks to make sure your last nine days are just as exciting as the first nine . . . minus the headaches, lethargy, and desire to tell co-workers happily eating donuts in the break room to shove it.

Melissa's Motivation

Habits are a fantastic brain adaptation. They let you manage chunks of your day with minimal effort, giving you more time, energy, and focus for the really important stuff. But it's easy to let your healthy Whole30 habits devolve into predictable, un-exciting, un-motivating practices. Now that your meal prep, emergency food management, and keeping-the-kitchen-clean routines are firmly in place, you can afford to put those habits on auto-pilot and take your focus and attention into other areas of your Whole30.

Yes, Whole30er . . . it's time to put in a little more effort. I know you've been working HARD, and you get all the high-fives for that, but if routine has you feeling down, a few small changes can make a world of difference. Over the next two days, we'll cover some tips to shake it off and get excited, because your Whole30 is about to go *next-level*.

FAQ

HOW CAN I GET OUT OF MY FOOD RUT? Having a few staple meals or eating the same basic breakfast template most mornings definitely makes things easier. But after a few weeks, what was comforting can become boring, leaving you uninspired and burned out. Here are two tricks for digging yourself out of a Whole30 meal rut.

➤ **TRY NEW FOODS.** Eggs are easy, and avocado and sweet potato are delicious, but there *are* other protein, fat, and carb sources. Start by trying a new vegetable or two—your local farmers market is a great place to score something fresh *and* get tips about how to prepare it. Or make the same food a new way—steamed green beans are exciting again when they're roasted in duck fat. Finally, new seasoning mixtures can really spice things up, turning your standard Mexi ground turkey into an Asian/Italian/Greek delight.

➤ **TRY NEW RECIPES.** This is where you get the most bang for your buck. Discovering a new favorite dish can energize your Whole30 for days! When Melissa's sister is feeling burned out, she'll text, "I'm OVER salmon cakes; need something new. Help?" Reaching out to someone with similar tastes or cooking preferences can make the recipe-finding job easier—or browse through *The Whole30*, *The Whole30 Cookbook*, *The Whole30 Fast & Easy Cookbook*, or @whole30recipes on Instagram for visual inspiration.

> **COMMUNITY INSPIRATION**
>
> "When you learn (more) about what foods work for you, it's easy to think, 'Why keep going, because I would love to have a glass of wine tonight . . . ' But I'm more than halfway through and learning new stuff every day. So when I think about quitting . . . mmm, better not." —*RantsFromMommyland.com*

TIP

If you've been making the same exact meals over and over, think about using meal templates instead of specific recipes. One of Melissa's favorites is "ground meat with stuff over stuff, topped with something." (She's thinking about trademarking it.) Here are three meals from that one template: 1. Ground beef, diced green peppers, onions, summer squash, and basil, over spaghetti squash, topped with tomato sauce. 2. Ground chicken, green onion, red pepper, and mushrooms, over zucchini noodles, topped with Yai's Thai Almond Sauce. 3. Ground lamb, grape tomatoes, diced cucumber, and mint, over baby spinach, topped with a homemade tzatziki sauce. Boom! Three *totally* different meals from the same template.

HACK

Any time you adopt a new habit, there's a balance to be found—jumping in with both feet can help you start off strong, but if you take on too much too soon, you'll get overwhelmed. Ask yourself, am I overcomplicating my Whole30? If you spend 30 minutes a day searching for new recipes, cook something brand-new every night, or make everything by hand (when convenience versions are easily accessible), maybe it's time to relax *instead* of kicking things up a notch. Give yourself a break from making an Instagram-worthy dinner; throw burgers and mixed veggies on the grill and serve with a side of Primal Kitchen Ranch. This will taste delicious *and* give you more time to enjoy all of the benefits your Whole30 has to offer.

EXTRA CREDIT: Get ready to dazzle your taste buds with some fresh new Whole30 meals. Choose a new recipe, scope the grocery store for new compliant ingredients, or relax a little, toss some leftovers on a paper plate, and use the hour you would have spent preparing dinner to do something fun!

It's almost like you're back where you started on Day 1, thinking so much about your Whole30 food! But this time, you're way more comfortable in your healthy habits, and taking on new food challenges from a place of excitement and confidence. So do your Extra Credit, but don't let it keep you from documenting all those NSVs! You've earned every single one.

What went well today: ....

....

....

....

What could have gone better: ....

....

....

....

What I'll do tomorrow: ....

....

....

....

Today's Extra Credit: ....

....

....

....

....

....

....

Today's NSVs

Energy

The Worst   The Best!

1   2   3   4   5   6   7   8   9   10

NOTES: ....

....

Sleep Quality

The Worst   The Best!

1   2   3   4   5   6   7   8   9   10

NOTES: ....

....

Cravings

The Worst   The Best!

1   2   3   4   5   6   7   8   9   10

NOTES: ....

....

FILL IN YOUR OWN

NSV #1: ....

....

....

NSV #2: ....

....

....

NSV #3: ....

....

....

WHAT I ATE

Favorite!

☐ Meal 1:..
....
....

☐ Meal 2:..
....
....

☐ Meal 3:..
....
....

Extra meal/snack:..
....
....

Day 21 Reflections

....
....
....
....
....
....
....

☐ **I did it! Whole30 Day 21 is in the bag.**

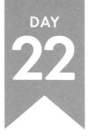

DAY 22

DAY 22 might have you feeling more inspired, energized, and motivated, especially after completing last night's Extra Credit and eating a delicious, all-new (probably egg-free) breakfast. But despite the tips we gave you on Day 15, are you still playing it cautious in your social life?

In the beginning, it's common and probably even helpful to decline social invitations with a lot of unknowns—who'll be there, what they'll be eating, and how much peer pressure you might face. At that stage in your Whole30 journey, it's more important to solidify your commitment and groove new habits than risk caving to temptation. But now you're more than three weeks in, and playing it safe will only hurt your cause. The Whole30 is designed to jump start a whole new lifestyle, and that has to include socializing! If you've been feeling left out or isolated during your program, put on your party pants, because that's all about to change.

Melissa's Motivation

You know the saying, "Fake it 'til you make it"? That applies here too, especially in unfamiliar social situations. You fear being the only one who orders with a million substitutions, drinks water at the baseball game, or passes on the birthday cake at work. You're confident in your Whole30 choices, but outside of friends and family, you feel less sure of yourself. So . . . *fake it*.

Fake ordering your substitutions with the utmost certainty and a huge smile. Fake patience and humor when refusing the offer of a beer for the sixth time. Fake being totally at ease when saying, "No thanks, I'm good" when the cake is passed your way. The more confident and comfortable you are in your Whole30 choices, the more easily your social partners will accept them, making you more likely to get out there and socialize.

FAQ

WHAT'S THE BEST WAY TO HANDLE SOCIAL SITUATION UNKNOWNS? Reviewing the menu, talking to the host ahead of time, or bringing your own dish are great, but mentally preparing is the real key to success.

➤ **IF/THEN PLANS.** Think about the challenges you might face, and create a plan for handling them. The more situations you can imagine, the better prepared you'll be! Consider questions you may get from family and friends ("If people ask what my weird diet is about, then . . ."), what you'll do if there is little you can eat ("If I'm not sure of the menu, then . . ."), how you'll deal with peer pressure ("If my co-worker insists I have a beer, then . . ."), and how you'll respond if someone takes your refusal of a dish personally ("If my host seems upset that I'm not trying her cheesecake, then . . .")

➤ **READ FOOD FREEDOM FOREVER.** You've started prepping for life after your Whole30 with *FFF*, but there are also three chapters devoted to talking to friends, family, and co-workers about food, including sample conversations to help you prepare for any social challenge. You don't have to steal our lines, but use the tips to create your own answers to tough questions . . . and then practice! Just as with social settings, the more confident and comfortable you are in your response, the faster other people will accept your choices and move on.

> **COMMUNITY INSPIRATION**
>
> "I am feeling good today! In my first Whole30, I didn't think I could handle going out to eat. This time, I have shown myself that I can dine out *and* make healthy choices. I've learned I don't have to stuff my face with high-calorie food to have a good time with my friends." —*Julie A., Ohio*

147

📌 TIP

The more you can take control of your socializing, the easier it will be to stick to the Whole30. Plus, people generally appreciate when you step up and take responsibility for coordinating events. If your group isn't sure where to dine, suggest a restaurant where it's easy to stay compliant; offer to host the first book club meeting; or invite the new boss to *your* house for dinner instead of going hers. And if you're dining at someone else's house, offering to bring a dish or two is almost always welcomed, especially if you explain to the host ahead of time you're doing a 30-day experiment to help you identify food sensitivities, and your diet is kind of particular right now.

HACK

Being confident in social situations is about a lot more than just your words; your body language speaks volumes. Part of "faking it" in stressful situations is appearing at ease using bodily cues that convey comfort, assuredness, and warmth. First, smile! The power of "No, thank you" PLUS a smile is magical. Make eye contact, stand or sit up straight with arms relaxed and open (not crossed in front of you), and don't apologize for your "weird order" or lack of participation in the beer/pizza/cake-fest. Asking a thoughtful question is also a powerful social tool, getting you out of repeated "What's this crazy diet again?" conversations while showing your partner that you're a good listener and interested in them.

EXTRA CREDIT: Make if/then plans for the coming week, identifying opportunities for (or creating) social situations where you can both enjoy the fun and stay Whole30 compliant. Review your talking points, watch a TED Talk on body language and confidence, and then practice as much as you can!

We're taking your Whole30 up a notch, but at this point in your journey, you're ready for some new challenges and the big rewards to follow. This life-changing stuff is hard, but you're committed and firmly entrenched in your growth mind-set. Prove it by finding at least one NSV that's changed for the better this week due to your hard work, perseverance, and belief in yourself.

22

What went well today: ....

....

....

....

What could have gone better: ....

....

....

....

What I'll do tomorrow: ....

....

....

....

Today's Extra Credit: ....

....

....

....

....

....

Today's NSVs

Energy

The Worst   The Best!

1   2   3   4   5   6   7   8   9   10

NOTES: ....

....

Sleep Quality

The Worst   The Best!

1   2   3   4   5   6   7   8   9   10

NOTES: ....

....

Cravings

The Worst   The Best!

1   2   3   4   5   6   7   8   9   10

NOTES: ....

....

FILL IN YOUR OWN

NSV #1: ....

....

....

NSV #2: ....

....

....

NSV #3: ....

....

....

WHAT I ATE

Favorite!

☐ Meal 1: ....
....
....

☐ Meal 2: ....
....
....

☐ Meal 3: ....
....
....
....

Extra meal/snack: ....
....
....

Day 22 Reflections

....
....
....
....
....
....
....

☐ **I did it! Whole30 Day 22 is in the bag.**

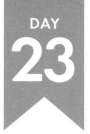

DAY

23

DAY 23 and you woke up feeling normal. But, like, NEW normal. Energized, happy, healthy normal. You're not even thinking about being on the Whole30, you're just thinking, THIS FEELS GOOD. You bop into the bathroom ready to dominate your day when you're met with the overwhelming urge to step on your scale. Or rescue your scale from the garage. Or saunter over to the neighbor's and casually ask, "Hey, do you guys have a scale?" Because today, YOU MUST KNOW.

The scale (and the mirror, and the selfie comparisons) are tempting in the last week of the program. Maybe it's because you've seen so many changes and you just want to quantify them, or you used to weigh daily and three weeks is a long time to go without, or because the instant gratification would feel good after three-plus weeks without food-related instant reward. Whatever the reason, *you will resist.* Read on.

🛟 Melissa's Motivation

You are doing AWESOME, and your Whole30 results are reflecting all of your hard work, consistency, and self-love. You feel amazing. You look fantastic. Self-confidence is through the roof. You're practically glowing, and people in your life are asking, "What have you been *doing*?" You *know* this is working. You're beginning to understand that this is just the start of your forever lifestyle, which is really exciting. And you know deep down inside that your scale will not serve you here.

It's just a number (and not a very telling one at that), and expectations are the thief of Whole30 joy. Ignore the echo of the scale, whispering that your self-worth, value, or success is dependent on the number. Right here and now, you can decide that it no longer has power over you. You've worked so hard. You've come so far. And you are *not* going out to a $20 hunk of plastic with just one week to go.

FAQ

I GET IT . . . BUT I STILL WANT TO LOSE WEIGHT. ANY TIPS?
We know you want to lose weight; we just want you to do it the right way. Our advice has nothing to do with counting calories, cutting carbs or fat, or killing yourself with exercise, because you've done that, and it's NEVER worked long-term.

→ **SLEEP.** We talked about sleep in Day 18, but this is perhaps the biggest unrecognized factor in body composition, aside from stress . . . and lack of sleep is stressful! (Double-whammy.)

→ **WALK.** Walking is the most underrated form of exercise for weight loss. Walk regularly, at a brisk pace. Maybe sometimes up a hill. Maybe sometimes with a backpack. Ideally outside in a green space. Hey, bring a friend!

→ **REDUCE STRESS.** Easier said than done, but we've got a strategy outlined in *Food Freedom Forever*, and remember the 20-minute stress/craving connection video mentioned in Day 6? That'll get you started.

→ **GROWTH MIND-SET.** The best thing you could do for your body composition long-term is stay connected to the idea that you are a healthy person, living a healthy lifestyle, surrounding yourself with people, places, things, and experiences to support that.

COMMUNITY INSPIRATION

"I'm feeling good! My last round I could not handle not weighing myself, but this round I'm not touching the scale and have been *amazed* at what a difference it makes! I'm eating based on when I'm hungry, and not (eating) less because I 'haven't lost weight.'"
—*Becca W., Colorado*

TIP

You may be tempted to "play" with your Whole30 at this point in your journey, throwing in intermittent fasting, a ketogenic approach, or timing macronutrients to see how your body reacts. This kind of self-experimentation can be instrumental in helping you create the perfect long-term diet for you . . . but smack in the middle of another self-experiment is NOT the time. The Whole30 is such a powerful protocol that you'll want to complete 30 days exactly as recommended and evaluate the results *before* throwing in additional factors. Once your program is over and you have a healthy baseline established, then you can play around with fasting, macronutrient timing, or calories to see whether that might benefit your health and fitness.

HACK

If there is ONE practice that we'd recommend to reduce stress, reinforce your growth mind-set, and help you achieve a healthy body composition, it's meditation . . . but not the sitting-in-lotus-for-an-hour kind. The mindful kind, done while conducting everyday tasks like working, talking with a friend, and eating. Being more aware of your food, conversation, or surroundings brings a sense of calm, helps you stay in touch with your body, and reduces the urge to "numb" with less healthy behaviors due to stress or anxiety. Mindful meditation also sends powerful signals to the body, helping you rest, digest your food, and reduce stress hormone levels. Visit mindful.org/meditation to learn how to take mindfulness into walks, conversations, or your bedtime routine.

EXTRA CREDIT: Practice mindfulness during dinner, get outside and go for a walk, or pick up an extra hour of sleep tonight (Facebook can wait). Oh, and if you haven't already, pre-commit and get that scale out of your bathroom!

After today, you're really starting to think about the "end" being in sight . . . but tomorrow we'll explain that this is really just the beginning of a whole new forever lifestyle. Take tonight to reflect on how far you've come, hitting those NSVs hard to remind yourself that your worth, values, and efforts are way more than just a number.

What went well today: _____

_____

_____

_____

What could have gone better: _____

_____

_____

_____

What I'll do tomorrow: _____

_____

_____

_____

Today's Extra Credit: _____

_____

_____

_____

_____

_____

Today's NSVs

Energy

The Worst   The Best!

1   2   3   4   5   6   7   8   9   10

NOTES: ....

....

Sleep Quality

The Worst   The Best!

1   2   3   4   5   6   7   8   9   10

NOTES: ....

....

Cravings

The Worst   The Best!

1   2   3   4   5   6   7   8   9   10

NOTES: ....

....

FILL IN YOUR OWN

NSV #1: ....

....

....

NSV #2: ....

....

....

NSV #3: ....

....

....

156

WHAT I ATE

Favorite!

☐ Meal 1: ....

....

....

....

☐ Meal 2: ....

....

....

....

☐ Meal 3: ....

....

....

....

Extra meal/snack: ....

....

....

Day 23 Reflections

....

....

....

....

....

....

☐ **I did it! Whole30 Day 23 is in the bag.**

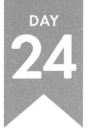

DAY
24

IT'S DAY 24... but if it weren't for this handbook, you'd have lost count by now. Your Whole30 is flying by, feeling totally natural at this point. Yay, life-changing! Except *somewhere* in the back of your head, you know Day 30 approacheth. Kinda soon, in fact. And if you stopped to think about it, *that* means your Whole30 is almost over. Finished. The end.

But as we'll explain, that train of thought can be an express journey straight into Cravingtown (Population: You)... so let's not think about it that way! Today is all about focusing on the *process* and not a defined "end." Remember, this isn't a diet—which means that even though there is a Day 31, there is no "end" where you're unceremoniously dumped right back into your old habits, lethargy, cravings, and waistline. The Whole30 is the first step on the lifelong path of discovering food freedom; a process that you'll happily embrace, refine, and enjoy for the rest of your life.

Melissa's Motivation

The Whole30 is just the first step in a lifelong journey of discovering your food freedom. You won't have to eat like this forever, and some of your old favorites may make the cut back into your regular healthy eating plan... but if you really want a healthy, sustainable, rewarding diet that will bring you a lifetime of benefits, you *will* have to continue practicing mindfulness, awareness, and conscientiousness around food for the rest of your life.

Really, though, this is excellent news! That means you have your *whole life* to play around with your own perfect diet, figure out how much wine/cheese/chocolate you can "get away with," and solidify the new, healthy habits that keep you looking and feeling your best. So if you've been thinking about the Whole30 "ending," reframe! This is just the first step, and it only gets better.

FAQ ◀—

24

HEY MELISSA, HOW DO YOU EAT WHEN YOU'RE NOT ON WHOLE30? If you're looking for a prescription (here's what I do, so you should do it too), you're not going to find that here. ME telling YOU what to eat isn't food freedom! What I *can* tell you is how I've used the Whole30 to think about my "life after" diet.

—▶ NO AND YES FOODS. During my elimination and reintroduction, I identified a few foods that are never worth it, based on how awful they made me feel when I brought them back in. (I'm looking at you, soft cheeses.) So I *never* eat those, because I never want to deal with the resulting "alien in the belly" feeling again. For other stuff, I noticed zero negative effects upon reintroduction, so I eat white rice on my sushi and hummus with my carrots regularly. I also observed that added sugar in condiments or meat sticks doesn't fire up my Sugar Dragon, so I don't worry about Honey Mustard salad dressing or date syrup in my jerky.

—▶ SOMETIMES FOODS. There are other foods (like bread, my mom's hermit cookies, or ice cream) that are maybe sometimes worth it, but they had better be REALLY good, and I had better be prepared to accept the resulting digestive distress, brain fog, and sugar cravings. I eat those when I choose, but always carefully and deliberately, keeping in mind that the less I eat, the better I'll feel.

> COMMUNITY INSPIRATION
>
> "I am currently in my fourth round with food freedom/Paleo living between rounds. When I started in September 2016, I was 60 pounds heavier. I have reversed my type 2 diabetes. No more meds and amazing A1c results. I am a card-carrying member of the Whole30 faithful."   —*Terry G., British Columbia*

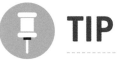

TIP

Your brain may be jumping ahead to Day 31, but you still have six days to go—and getting complacent at this point can spell trouble. Food boredom, "25 is just as good as 30," and "I've been so good, I deserve a treat" may come creeping in, tempting you to compromise your commitment. Don't go there! It's good to plan ahead, but commit to making the last week of Whole30 your best one yet. Take advantage of your Tiger Blood and do something fitness-y, find new recipes to make the next six days of dinner extra-exciting, and proactively treat yo'self . . . with one of the *non-food-related rewards* you identified in Day 10. Don't get lazy now—for many, this last week brings even MORE magic, but only if you keep actively working the program.

HACK

Habit research (done with flight attendants who smoked cigarettes) shows that when your brain perceives reward on the horizon, cravings come back with a vengeance. This partially explains why people binge hard after coming off a short-term weight loss diet . . . the diet is "over," so the brain wants everything you've been denying it, all at once! That's why it's important NOT to think about your Whole30 as "ending," just transitioning into the next phase. It's one long cycle, each step building on the last, with a robust support system built into each phase. So tell your brain, "Calm down . . . nothing's *over*! We're just gonna keep rolling with all of these amazing benefits and delicious, satisfying foods."

EXTRA CREDIT: Write down three ways you can ENERGIZE your Whole30 in the last few days. Ideas: start reading/listening to *Food Freedom Forever* (more on this in Day 29), find some new recipes, have a "home stretch" celebratory dinner party, or pick up that kitchen gadget you've been eyeing.

Transfer your newfound Whole30 energy into tonight's reflections, spending extra time focusing on what went well today, and what you're going to do tomorrow to finish your Whole30 strong. Consider going back through past reflections and bringing some of your "favorited" meals back into rotation, too!

24

What went well today: ....

....

....

....

....

What could have gone better: ....

....

....

....

....

What I'll do tomorrow: ....

....

....

....

....

Today's Extra Credit: ....

....

....

....

....

....

....

....

Today's NSVs

Energy

The Worst   The Best!

1   2   3   4   5   6   7   8   9   10

NOTES: ....

....

Sleep Quality

The Worst   The Best!

1   2   3   4   5   6   7   8   9   10

NOTES: ....

....

Cravings

The Worst   The Best!

1   2   3   4   5   6   7   8   9   10

NOTES: ....

....

FILL IN YOUR OWN

NSV #1: ....

....

NSV #2: ....

....

NSV #3: ....

....

WHAT I ATE

Favorite!

☐ Meal 1:..
....
....

☐ Meal 2:..
....
....

☐ Meal 3:..
....
....

Extra meal/snack:..
....
....

Day 24 Reflections

....
....
....
....
....
....
....

☐ **I did it! Whole30 Day 24 is in the bag.**

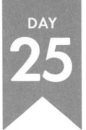

DAY

25

HAPPY DAY 25! Your Whole30 is bright and shiny again, and you're fully committed to finishing strong. In fact, you're feeling SO good and things are going SO well that you're wondering if you should make it a Whole40 or Whole60.

It's common for people to consider extending their program at this point in the journey. We'll help you figure out if extending your Whole30 is right for you, but you don't have to decide right this minute. In fact, between now and Day 30, you'll probably vacillate between "I could do this forever!" and "I can't wait to reintroduce." So don't make any hasty decisions—you've got five more days to figure it out. In the meantime, enjoy your Tiger Blood, be supported by the structure of the rules, and see what additional benefits you can wring out of your Whole30.

Melissa's Motivation

Some of you might be nervous about Day 31, wondering whether a Whole-Forever is actually a viable option. There are a number of reasons you'd want to extend your program, but being afraid to let go of the rules or eat something not-Whole30 isn't one of them. Remember, we haven't eliminated these foods from the program because they're BAD, we've eliminated them because they're UNKNOWN (and often problematic). The whole experiment is designed to help you figure out how these foods work for you, so you can bring your choice of delicious, special, or culturally-relevant foods back into your life in a way that works for you.

Staying on the program out of fear of eating something off-plan or having to create your own guidelines is NOT food freedom. The point of the Whole30 is to jump-start a whole new lifestyle, where YOU make the food-related decisions that are right for you. And the only way to arrive at that place is to *practice*.

FAQ

←

HOW DO I KNOW IF EXTENDING MY WHOLE30 IS RIGHT FOR ME? If you're in one of these categories, you may want to consider adding some days.

→ **MEDICAL CONDITIONS.** If you have a longstanding medical condition, especially chronic pain, fatigue, or an autoimmune illness, 30 days probably isn't long enough to see the most dramatic changes the program could offer. If you're already seeing an improvement in symptoms, that's a good indicator that more time could bring you more relief. Consult your healthcare provider first, to make sure extending is recommended for you.

→ **FOOD "ADDICTIONS."** If you've got a long history with serious cravings or consider yourself a sugar/carb addict, you may want to stay on the Whole30 until you feel totally in control and ready to reintroduce potentially triggering foods. If you're working with a counselor, speak with them about your progress and this decision, and follow their advice.

→ **STRESSFUL EVENTS.** If you've got a stressful but short-term event during or just after Day 31, like a presentation at work or a family visit, staying on the program through this time period can help you keep calm and focused, and reduces the risk that stress will drive you right back into old comfort habits and hijack your planned reintroduction.

COMMUNITY INSPIRATION

"I'm going to keep going for at least 60 days. I feel pretty amazing! My arthritic hands don't hurt anymore! All my aches and pains are gone! I know that I have all the tools I need to be successful at this. It's 100% up to me." —*Jennifer M., Florida*

TIP

If you're planning to extend your Whole30, you'd better be prepared! While you've got the food planning and prep part down by now, you'll face new challenges starting on Day 31. Food boredom is a real danger, so keep your list of favorite meals from your daily reflections handy, and make the effort to find new recipes. Stay social; both for the support and to show friends this new lifestyle isn't going to create distance in your relationships. Finally, practice your elevator pitch for when people ask you why you're STILL on this "crazy diet," generously detailing the benefits you've seen and the specific reasons you think extending your program is right for you.

HACK

You've created and enforced new, healthy habits over the last 25 days, and you'd think after this long, the old draw to the pantry after dinner or automatic reach for a wine glass after a tough day at work would be gone. But habit research shows that, on average, it takes 66 days for a new habit to stick, and that old habits never really go away—they're just overwritten by new ones. If you're still experiencing the pull of an old habit, don't let it throw you. When you're tired, stressed, or distracted, the brain is more likely to gravitate toward old comforting routines—and since your connection to food is pretty emotional, it may take longer to break those old ties. Just be aware when the cues come up, and purposefully transition to your new practice or reward. Consistency is key.

EXTRA CREDIT: If you're going to extend your Whole30, set some goals, consider a timeline (how many days will you add?), and make the plans outlined in the Tip. If you're going to do the 30 as prescribed, brush up on the Reintroduction chapter and FAQ in *The Whole30*.

With only five days to go, you may be tempted to start slacking in your reflections. Please don't! Staying connected to the process here will help you stay motivated right up until the end. More important, you'll want the details to help you compare your first week to your last, and (thinking ahead) to compare your next Whole30 experience to this one.

What went well today: ....

....

....

....

....

What could have gone better: ....

....

....

....

What I'll do tomorrow: ....

....

....

....

....

Today's Extra Credit: ....

....

....

....

....

....

....

25

Today's NSVs

Energy

The Worst   The Best!

1   2   3   4   5   6   7   8   9   10

NOTES: ....

....

Sleep Quality

The Worst   The Best!

1   2   3   4   5   6   7   8   9   10

NOTES: ....

....

Cravings

The Worst   The Best!

1   2   3   4   5   6   7   8   9   10

NOTES: ....

....

FILL IN YOUR OWN

NSV #1: ....

....

....

NSV #2: ....

....

....

NSV #3: ....

....

....

WHAT I ATE

Favorite!

☐ Meal 1: ....

....

....

....

☐ Meal 2: ....

....

....

....

☐ Meal 3: ....

....

....

....

Extra meal/snack: ....

....

....

25

Day 25 Reflections

....

....

....

....

....

....

☐ **I did it! Whole30 Day 25 is in the bag.**

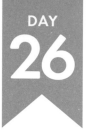

HEY HEY, DAY 26 . . . and what a great day it is, with Tiger Blood in full effect! Whether or not you'll extend your Whole30 journey, you're definitely thinking about what your reintroduction will look like. How many days will it take? What if you don't *want* to reintroduce something? What kind of symptoms can you expect if you reintroduce something to which you are sensitive?

Now that your Whole30 is mostly on auto-pilot, you've got some capacity to start thinking about "life after," and the first phase of *that* is your 10-plus day reintroduction period. While everything you need is found in *The Whole30*, we'll give you a high-level view here to help you plan and prepare.

Melissa's Motivation

Today, before we discuss next steps or "life after," I want you to think about how the Whole30 has changed you. Not physically—although it certainly has. Not your habits, although you've created plenty of new ones, and dropped some that weren't serving you. But how has the Whole30 changed you *as a person*? Strange, maybe, to think about a short-term dietary protocol as having truly life-changing potential, and yet the Whole30 has the power to do just that—as you're probably well aware by now. So how has it changed *you*?

You're less anxious, or calmer in general. You handle stress more gracefully, and have more presence and control when faced with difficult things. You feel closer to your partner, best friend, or children. You're more focused, productive, and creative. Your self-confidence is evident in your posture, your smile, your willingness to engage with the world. You're brave and bold, trying things you've always wanted to try. This is YOUR life-changing Whole30 experience. And you should be so proud of every last one of these positive changes you've made in your life.

FAQ

WHAT'S THE DIFFERENCE BETWEEN THE TWO REINTRO-DUCTION OPTIONS? *The Whole30* outlines two different protocols for reintroduction: Fast Track and Slow Roll. Here's the difference:

→ **FAST TRACK.** In this protocol, you reintroduce all of the food groups within a 10-day period (14 with alcohol). You'll reintro in the order of *least* likely to be problematic to *most* likely to be problematic, going back to the Whole30 for two days between reintroduction groups. This is perfect for those who want to begin their food freedom as soon as possible, but may make for a not-so-pleasant 10 days, if it turns out you're sensitive to multiple food groups.

→ **SLOW ROLL.** Come Day 31, you'll give yourself some breathing room by relaxing on the "no added sugar" rule for things like meat and condiments, but maintain a Whole30-ish diet until something SO special and tempting comes along that you decide you want to reintroduce just that one food (regardless of the food group it's in). This allows you to retain your Whole30 Tiger Blood while bringing foods back in slowly and discriminately. If you've seen a huge improvement in autoimmune or chronic pain or fatigue symptoms and fear a 10-day reintroduction may compromise your quality of life tremendously, the Slow Roll is for you.

26

"I'm on Day 26 and started feeling an inner peace about a week ago that I can't put into words. My anxiety has lifted, the sun is shining brighter, and my soul feels refreshed. Thank you for this experience. It has truly been life-changing."

—*Mary L., Minnesota*

📌 TIP

If you don't miss a particular food, don't bother reintroducing it! Reintroduction is supposed to teach you which of your favorite foods you can bring back into your diet in a way that feels rewarding and sustainable, but keeps you looking and feeling your best. If you see no reason to ever go back to peanut butter, skip it! If you change your mind later, you can always reintroduce it in your food freedom or after your next reset. The only exception is something you want to test just in case you're accidentally exposed, like gluten. You may choose not to include gluten in your daily diet, but want to know what happens if you accidentally eat it in a restaurant—so reintroduction here might be smart.

HACK

You may be tempted to reintroduce "Paleo" versions of your favorite treats (like pancakes, banana bread, or cereal) more casually than gluten-grains; as their ingredients are mostly Whole30 compliant, what can it hurt? Proceed with caution, though, because after a month without your favorite comfort foods, your brain won't differentiate between an almond flour pancake and the real deal—and these sweets and treats may wake your Sugar Dragon fast and hard. If you want to test these foods, go for it, but separate them out from the rest of your reintroduction protocol and practice brutal self-awareness in the following days. These foods may not physically affect you as hard as real grains would, but if they impact cravings, energy, or mood, that's worth paying attention to.

EXTRA CREDIT: Guided by the Reintroduction chapter (page 42) and FAQ (page 132) in *The Whole30*, write down a general plan (Fast Track vs. Slow Roll, separating out alcohol or sugar, other foods you want to test separately, etc.) for Day 31.

To help plan for reintroduction, focus on all of the benefits you've seen so far, emphasizing the ones you refuse to live without now that you know you can look and feel *this* good. Mark these NSVs with a star, and don't be afraid to star a LOT! These markers will help you evaluate whether a reintroduced food is *really* worth it in your food freedom.

What went well today: ....

....

....

....

....

What could have gone better: ....

....

....

....

....

What I'll do tomorrow: ....

....

....

....

....

Today's Extra Credit:..

....

....

....

....

....

....

26

Today's NSVs

Energy

The Worst   The Best!

1   2   3   4   5   6   7   8   9   10

NOTES: ....

....

Sleep Quality

The Worst   The Best!

1   2   3   4   5   6   7   8   9   10

NOTES: ....

....

Cravings

The Worst   The Best!

1   2   3   4   5   6   7   8   9   10

NOTES: ....

....

FILL IN YOUR OWN

NSV #1: ....

....

....

NSV #2: ....

....

....

NSV #3: ....

....

....

WHAT I ATE

Favorite!

☐ Meal 1: ....
....
....

☐ Meal 2: ....
....
....

☐ Meal 3: ....
....
....

Extra meal/snack: ....
....
....

Day 26 Reflections

....
....
....
....
....
....
....

☐ **I did it! Whole30 Day 26 is in the bag.**

GOOD MORNING, DAY 27! Allow us to be repetitive ... you feel awesome. You look awesome. Life is good! But you're probably *still* a little nervous about what your reintroduction period will bring. What if it sends you off the rails? What if it your asthma returns? What if you bring your beloved diet soda back ... and you don't even like it anymore?

The last few days of your Whole30 journey is a lot like the first few—equal parts excitement and trepidation. You're excited for the next phase but worried that reintroducing anything new will knock you off your Tiger Blood. Don't be a scaredy-cat ... while there may be unpleasant parts, reintroduction can be really fun, and we'll give you all the tips you'll need to retain your desired Whole30 benefits along the way.

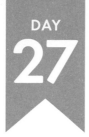 **Melissa's Motivation**

You may be worried that eating bread, wine, cheese, or sugar again will instantly ruin all the progress you've made; sending you back into the same unhealthy spiral of craving, overconsumption, and stress, or undoing all of the health benefits or symptom improvements you've seen. Please don't worry—we'll support you here, too.

First, we've built a buffer right into our reintroduction schedule, so if you *do* eat something that throws you psychologically, going right back to the Whole30 for two days will keep you on track. Second, you've healed your body from the inside out for 30 days in a row—that progress can't be wiped out with a day of bread or cheese! You may have a rough experience, but another few days of Whole30 will bring you right back to Tiger Blood, helping you figure out how much and how often you may be able to eat that food while still looking and feeling awesome. It's all a learning experience, but if at any point you feel out of sorts, just return to the Whole30 until you're solid again.

FAQ

DO I REALLY NEED TO DO 10 MORE DAYS OF NEAR-WHOLE30 EATING? As mentioned, there's a buffer built into our reintroduction schedule (a few days of Whole30 between reintro food groups). And yes, you have to do it.

LEARN. The only way you'll know how a reintroduced food impacts you physically or emotionally is to reintroduce JUST that food back into your Whole30 diet. Think of it like a scientific experiment, where the Whole30 is the "control" and the reintroduced food is the experimental factor. If you bring pizza, beer, and ice cream back all at once, you'll never know what to blame for the foggy brain, upset stomach, energy crash, or joint pain. That means your meals on reintroduction days will look mostly Whole30, plus just one added off-plan ingredient or food to evaluate.

RESET. Not every reintroduced food will bring on immediate digestive distress or lethargy. It may take a day or two to notice joint inflammation, skin breakouts, the return of aches or pains, or other physical symptoms. Returning to the Whole30 after each reintro day helps you better evaluate the true impact of that food group. It also allows your system calm down between food groups, keeping any negative side effects from piling up and confusing your evaluation process ("My skin broke out; was that today's bread or yesterday's milk?").

27

COMMUNITY INSPIRATION

"Seeing a ton of NSVs and feeling great. Nervous about 'falling off the wagon' once the 30 days are done. Trying to focus on the overarching lifestyle changes I want to make, rather than seeing this as a 30-day event. I'm speed-reading *Food Freedom Forever* so I can form a plan." —*Kelsey T., Facebook*

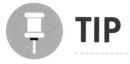

TIP

As mentioned, one reason we give you Whole30 days between reintroduction days is to protect you against cravings or emotional eating. There's also a good chance that something you'll eat during reintroduction will bring up old diet-thinking known as the *What the Hell Effect*: "I've already ruined my diet, might as well eat this stuff too." Knowing you're going back to the comfort and security of the Whole30 rules for a few days derails that train of thought, and gives you the confidence to try things that you suspect might be problematic but still want to test. Think of it as a shield against your fire-breathing Sugar Dragon, should one of your reintro choices stir him up.

HACK

Habit research says that black-and-white rules are easier for the brain to follow, taking some of the decision-making process out of your "willpower center" and moving it into "habit territory." You've probably already experienced this during your Whole30, automatically turning down alcohol or reading a product label. The idea of losing those parameters may feel scary, but don't be nervous! Making your own decisions during the safety net of reintroduction is a great way to practice riding your own bike. Knowing you'll be back to the black-and-white rules between every reintroduction food group will free you to *really* test-drive the stuff you've been missing—and learn as much as you can about how it works for you.

EXTRA CREDIT: If you're already feeling guilty about consuming beer, cheese, or chocolate again, re-read page 61 in *Food Freedom Forever*. This section emphasizes that there is no guilt or shame in reintroducing off-plan foods—in fact, bringing this stuff back is a valuable and necessary part of the learning experience.

It's the final days of your Whole30, and while we're talking a lot about what your next steps will look like, there is still a lot to be gleaned from today's Whole30 experience. You never know what day something will finally "click," so if you had an a-ha moment, noticed a new NSV, or casually rocked something that used to feel hard, high-five yourself and detail it here.

What went well today: ....

....

....

....

....

What could have gone better: ....

....

....

....

....

What I'll do tomorrow: ....

....

....

....

....

Today's Extra Credit: ....

....

....

....

....

....

....

27

Today's NSVs

Energy

The Worst   The Best!

1   2   3   4   5   6   7   8   9   10

NOTES: ....

....

Sleep Quality

The Worst   The Best!

1   2   3   4   5   6   7   8   9   10

NOTES: ....

....

Cravings

The Worst   The Best!

1   2   3   4   5   6   7   8   9   10

NOTES: ....

....

FILL IN YOUR OWN

NSV #1: ....

....

....

NSV #2: ....

....

....

NSV #3: ....

....

....

WHAT I ATE

Favorite!

☐ Meal 1: ....

....

....

....

☐ Meal 2: ....

....

....

....

☐ Meal 3: ....

....

....

....

Extra meal/snack: ....

....

....

Day 27 Reflections

....

....

....

....

....

....

....

☐ **I did it! Whole30 Day 27 is in the bag.**

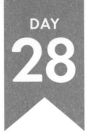

DAY
28

IT'S YOUR WHOLE30 DAY 28! Four weeks! T-minus 2 days and counting! You've pushed through the rough spots, fought off the food boredom, and love where you are right now. This Whole30 thing feels like second nature. Until you get to work, and your co-workers birthday cup-cakes SPEAK TO YOU. You've been so *good*. It's been so *long*. You're practically *done already*. Isn't 28 basically just as good as 30?

No, it's not. And this is the day—not 27, not 29, but Day 28—when people think about caving the most. It's the top of the roller coaster again; the last hill of the ride. You can almost see the end, but not quite . . . and bailing now could be disastrous for your self-confidence, cravings, and NSVs. (From way up here, it's a long way to fall.) So get that thought out of your head and use today's tips and motivation to see you through another delicious, rewarding day of Whole30.

Melissa's Motivation

Here's a little piece of tough love (heavy on the love) to start your day off right: you are *not* going out early; no way, no how. You made a commitment to give yourself 30 full days of good food and healthy habits. You made a commitment to finish the Whole30, and reintro-duce food in a systematic, deliberate fashion. You made a commit-ment to change your life, and the program you chose takes 30 days.

Take these promises seriously. If you cop out now, you're telling yourself the commitments you make to yourself are open to compro-mise, and that you're not important enough to honor your promise to yourself. But that is simply not true. You are important. You are worth the promises. And you *will* finish all 30 days. So take a deep breath, say, "No, thank you," and give yourself a gold star for seeing your commitment through. I promise it's much more satisfying than a store-bought cupcake.

FAQ

REMIND ME AGAIN WHY I'M NOT GOING TO REBOUND ON DAY 31? At this stage of your Whole30, it's common to see ghosts of dieting past: deprivation leading to bingeing leading to weight gain and "failure." But remember, this is not that.

NOT A DIET. The Whole30 isn't a quick-fix weight loss diet. You haven't starved. You haven't relied on willpower alone—you've successfully changed habits. You've also changed your tastes, blood sugar regulation, and hormonal balance, eliminating the "need sugar stat" signals and getting you back in touch with your body's own natural regulatory mechanisms. You're now effectively grounded in a healthy relationship with food *and* a healthy, balanced body.

YOU HAVE A PLAN. The 10-plus day reintroduction period is carefully designed to ease you into "riding your own bike," letting you bring back potentially less healthy foods at your discretion while surrounding you with the structure and comfort of the Whole30 rules. Once this tremendous learning period is over, you'll finally be armed with the knowledge to make the right decisions for yourself going forward, based on what you learn about how specific food groups affect you. No other diet has *ever* given you the information you need to create the perfect long-term diet for you—and that's a huge part of why things will be different this time.

28

COMMUNITY INSPIRATION

"I can't explain how amazing I feel. My momentum is at an all-time high. I used to be so sluggish that I just wanted to sleep all hours of the day. Now I feel motivated for LIFE. I have goals that feel so attainable now. This is my second Whole30, and it has been life-changing."   —*Joe S., Facebook*

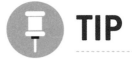

TIP

We're giving you a lot to think about here—your upcoming reintroduction, and (tomorrow) what your food freedom plan will look like post-reintro. But now is also a great time to think about how you can continue to support your new, healthy habits and growth mind-set when Day 31 rolls around. The best way to do this is to stay connected to the Whole30 community even after your program is over. You'll be able to offer support to new folks, inspire them with your Whole30 story and NSVs, and remind yourself through these connections that you are a healthy person living a healthy lifestyle. Surrounding yourself with so many health-minded, motivated, positive-thinking people will keep you inspired to work your food freedom plan!

HACK

Continuing today's "thinking ahead" theme, are there other areas in your life where the structure and black-and-white nature of the Whole30 could serve you—*and* support the idea that you are a healthy person with healthy habits? Melissa has a rule that she never goes to bed with a messy kitchen or dishes in the sink. No matter what, she cleans up in the evening . . . and reaps the benefits of feeling organized, in control, and calm in the morning when she walks into a tidy space. If you found the Whole30 structure effective, saying "ZERO dirty dishes" may be more effective in helping you maintain a neat home than saying, "I'll try to keep things clean" or "Just this once, I'll leave them."

EXTRA CREDIT: Using either the Tip or the Hack, choose just one area of focus (community connection or a healthy habit you'd like to create) during the reintroduction period and your food freedom. Outline a plan to reinforce your growth mind-set and keep you firmly entrenched in your new healthy lifestyle.

If today was a day of temptation, check off that "I did it!" box with a Sharpie and a smiley-face! If you used specific tips or tricks to distract or power through cravings, temptation, or peer pressure, highlight those here; you'll find those same tricks helpful in your food freedom. (And don't neglect your NSVs—we know you're still seeing them roll in.)

What went well today: ....

....

....

....

....

What could have gone better: ....

....

....

....

....

What I'll do tomorrow: ....

....

....

....

....

Today's Extra Credit: ....

....

....

....

....

....

....

28

Today's NSVs

Energy

The Worst   The Best!

1   2   3   4   5   6   7   8   9   10

NOTES: ....

....

Sleep Quality

The Worst   The Best!

1   2   3   4   5   6   7   8   9   10

NOTES: ....

....

Cravings

The Worst   The Best!

1   2   3   4   5   6   7   8   9   10

NOTES: ....

....

FILL IN YOUR OWN

NSV #1: ....

....

....

NSV #2: ....

....

....

NSV #3: ....

....

....

WHAT I ATE

Favorite!

☐ Meal 1: ....
....
....
....

☐ Meal 2: ....
....
....
....

☐ Meal 3: ....
....
....
....

Extra meal/snack: ....
....
....

Day 28 Reflections

28

☐ **I did it! Whole30 Day 28 is in the bag.**

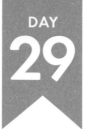

DAY 29, and you're WINNING your Whole30. Any thoughts you had of throwing in the towel early are *so* gone. You'll effortlessly cruise through this day, because tomorrow is Day 30! Wait. TOMORROW IS DAY 30.

Today's Timeline headline: HolyoprahitsalmostoverwhatamIgoingtoeatnow? But don't let this small thought grow into full-blown panic! You know we're supporting you with a carefully structured reintroduction period, but we also offer a complete "life after" guide in *Food Freedom Forever*. Like, the 3-step dietary plan you'll follow *for the rest of your life*. And while the Whole30 has brought you incredible life-changing benefits, you knew it was designed to be a short-term thing, not your forever lifestyle. So deep breath, because we (and *FFF*) are with you every step of the way.

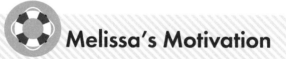

Melissa's Motivation

The phrase "food freedom" was born from post-Whole30 testimonials, in which graduates reported feeling happy, confident, and in control of their food for the first time in a long time. They said it felt like freedom; the freedom to eat a cookie and not beat yourself up, to enjoy vacation without punishing yourself when you got home, to say no to something that used to hold power over you, but no longer does. That is what *Food Freedom Forever* is all about, and that is what I want for you when your Whole30 is over.

Anyone can attain this sense of self-confidence, this place of balance, the feeling of being in control of your food for the first time in a long time, and I'll explain *exactly* how to do just that. I want you to feel just as supported in your food freedom journey as you did during your Whole30. You've been waiting your whole life for this, whether you realize it or not. You're almost ready to ride your own bike, and it's time to get excited for YOUR food freedom.

FAQ

HOW DOES *FOOD FREEDOM FOREVER* KEEP ME ON TRACK?
The 3-part Food Freedom plan is designed to run in a cycle, encouraging you to enjoy long periods of food freedom and return to the reset only when your habits start to slip. Plus, there are two additional ways *Food Freedom Forever* helps you stick to your new healthy lifestyle.

➤ **THE LANGUAGE OF FOOD.** *FFF* encourages you to lose the "diet" mentality, which makes you think that unless you're starving yourself or seriously restricting, you can't be healthy or lose weight. It also helps you change unhealthy thought patterns around food being "good" or "bad," and YOU being good or bad when you eat. Reframing how you look at food, your diet, and your body helps you break out of the yo-yo diet cycle and make true lifestyle changes.

➤ **FRIENDS AND FAMILY.** During the Whole30, it's easy to explain to friends and family why you're turning down beer, mom's cookies, or pizza—you're on the program, and the rules are strict. But when Day 31 rolls around and you STILL don't want the beer, cookies, or pizza, it may be harder to articulate your food freedom plan. *FFF* gives you three chapters dedicated to talking to friends, family, and co-workers about your reset and your food freedom, in a way that brings you closer together and helps you maintain your commitment to your own health.

COMMUNITY INSPIRATION

"I'm doing my second round of Whole30 while listening to *FFF* on Audible, and it is making all the pieces fit together so much more in my mind! It just makes sense, and has already alleviated so much of the stress I associated with reintroduction the first time around."   —*@candice_qh*

29

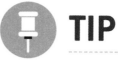

TIP

Now is a great time to start prepping your family and friends for the days to come. They may be thinking, "Sweet, on Day 31, I'll finally get my pancake brunch/wine on the patio/ice cream buddy back!" So have the conversation about the importance of reintroduction, the Whole30 benefits you've seen so far, and why you aren't willing to throw them all away for a pancake/wine/ice cream binge. This will allow them to better support you during reintroduction, and reduce the chance they'll try to peer-pressure you into cutting it short. Bonus: Use this time to arrange a date, family dinner, or celebration on one of your reintroduction days, combining your scheduled reintro foods with a fun social occasion!

HACK

Habit expert M.J. Ryan says having a slogan, mantra, or physical prompt can help you maintain the healthy habits you've established while on the Whole30. She suggests making them bold and specific; a concrete reminder of how to achieve the new goal. (And they don't have to mean anything to anyone besides you.) Bring a Whole30-stickered water bottle to office birthday parties to remind you to only eat the cake if it's worth it, tell yourself, "I'm an adult" when you're feeling peer pressure at happy hour, think, "Stay awake" when stress is tempting you to numb your feelings with food, or write "Tiger Blood > Sugar Dragon" on a Post-it and stick it to your fridge as a reminder that your inner Tiger is stronger than that pesky Dragon.

EXTRA CREDIT: Use this space to note key support people you're going to speak to before reintroduction, and what points you want to make in the conversation; OR choose a few healthy habits you want to reinforce, and create mantras or reminders to carry with you into your food freedom.

It's your second-to-last day of Whole30 reflections . . . but this day deserves your full attention just as much as any other. You might be amazed at the NSVs just popping up now, or how much more solid an existing NSV is feeling. Document it all, because you're really going to want to look back on these last few days with pride.

What went well today: ....

....

....

....

....

What could have gone better: ....

....

....

....

....

What I'll do tomorrow: ....

....

....

....

....

Today's Extra Credit:..

....

....

....

....

....

....

....

29

Today's NSVs

Energy

The Worst   The Best!

1   2   3   4   5   6   7   8   9   10

NOTES: ....

....

Sleep Quality

The Worst   The Best!

1   2   3   4   5   6   7   8   9   10

NOTES: ....

....

Cravings

The Worst   The Best!

1   2   3   4   5   6   7   8   9   10

NOTES: ....

....

FILL IN YOUR OWN

NSV #1: ....

....

....

NSV #2: ....

....

....

NSV #3: ....

....

....

WHAT I ATE

Favorite!

☐ Meal 1:..
....
....
....

☐ Meal 2:..
....
....
....

☐ Meal 3:..
....
....
....

Extra meal/snack:..
....
....

Day 29 Reflections

....
....
....
....
....
....
....

29

☐ **I did it! Whole30 Day 29 is in the bag.**

DAY

30

IT'S HERE, IT'S HERE . . . Whole30 Day 30!!! You did it, and we couldn't be any happier for you. You *feel* amazing. You *look* amazing. You can't stop grinning, and you just want to shout out to the whole world, "I FINISHED THE WHOLE30!" (Well, technically you might still have a few hours to go . . . but of course, you'll finish strong.)

Let the sense of self-confidence you feel right now carry over into every single part of your day. Stand tall, make eye contact, and smile a lot, because now more than ever, you KNOW that you can do hard things. (Oh, and you *should* announce your success to the whole world! We can even help with that, with graphics and a completion certificate you can download at whole30.com/i-finished-the-whole30/.)

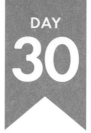 ## Melissa's Motivation

The only thing I want to say today is . . . YOU DID IT. You took on something that you knew would be hard and you worked on it every single day, with purpose and determination. You experienced plenty of challenges—some that made you wonder if you should just give up. Still, you did not quit. You struggled physically and emotionally, sometimes using sheer willpower or stubbornness to get through the day. Still, you did not quit. You faced social pressures, ranging from questions to teasing to downright hostility toward your "crazy diet." Still, you did not quit.

More than anything, remember this feeling. Remember the next time life is rough, you feel overwhelmed, or the outcome is uncertain; remember this one time that you took on something hard, and YOU DID NOT QUIT. This is who you are—a tough, capable, confident person who refused to give up on yourself; who wasn't afraid to ask for help; and who realized that in gracefully accepting support from others, you actually became *stronger*. This is who you are, and I am so proud of you.

FAQ

MY FRIENDS WANT TO HAVE A POST-WHOLE30 CELEBRATION. HOW CAN I DO THIS WITHOUT MESSING UP REINTRODUCTION? Here are two ideas for sharing your accomplishment with your support team while staying on track.

> **HOST A PARTY.** Have a dinner, barbecue, or brunch at your house (or let a friend host it for you), but make sure you have a hand in the menu. Work your first reintroduction food group into the mix, but keep the rest of your dishes Whole30-friendly. A tapas party or buffet is a great option here; you can have Whole30 dishes, non-compliant dishes for friends and family, and a reintroduction dish or two that overlaps with both groups.

> **SUGGEST A NON-FOOD-RELATED CELEBRATION.** You no longer believe rewarding yourself with junk food is much of a "treat," but your friends and family may feel defensive or judged if you say so out loud. Instead, tell them you'd love to celebrate, then suggest something active or community-related, like a group hike, getting tickets to a sporting event, a night of bowling or mini-golf, or an afternoon at the park or pool. It's YOUR party, after all, so you should get to choose what you do! Plus this scenario reinforces the idea that you don't need beer, cake, or chocolate to enjoy the company of those you love and celebrate your success.

COMMUNITY INSPIRATION

"I can see the light! My pain is gone. I can get out and move around without worrying about full body pain or migraines. Better sleep. No brain fog. I feel like this has finally clicked; like this lifestyle is actually doable. And I'm down 17 pounds and 16.5 inches! I'm so happy!!!"   —*Kara G., Minnesota*

30

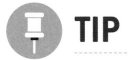

TIP

You *really* want to share your Whole30 efforts and results with the world . . . and here are three reasons why you should! *One*, your testimonial will remind people what the Whole30 is, and what it isn't. If people were skeptical of claims that this wasn't a fad or quick-fix weight loss plan, they won't be once they hear about your self-confidence gains and NSVs. *Two*, publicly proclaiming your success lets your support team share in the joy, and gives you an opportunity to thank each and every one of them for their contributions. *Three*, your energy, enthusiasm, and happiness will inspire others to change their lives with the Whole30 too, giving you the chance to give back by being there for *them* during their journey.

HACK

You may be tempted to wake up tomorrow and jump right on the scale . . . but is that really the right move for you? If you're at all anxious about the number that might appear, worried that if it's not small enough or doesn't meet your "goal," you'll feel like your Whole30 was a failure, DO NOT GET ON THE SCALE. Yes, it's tempting, and yes, you hope you've lost weight. But your Whole30 wasn't about weight loss, and it'd be a shame to let that $20 hunk of plastic override all of the amazing benefits and self-confidence you've gained. There's no harm in waiting, or not weighing at all if you think it'll take you to an unhealthy place. Use your NSV checklist, before-and-after photos, and the compliments of friends and family as proof that your Whole30 was a smashing success.

EXTRA CREDIT: Your Day 30 treat? Go back to the NSV checklist on page 16. How many of those accomplishments you marked as goals on Day 0 can you check off now? In fact, keep going down the list, checking ALL that apply. Be generous—you've worked hard for every last one!

Use tonight's reflections to heap praise upon yourself. Literally—gush. All of the good you've seen. All of the work you've done. The only thing you should be thinking today is, "I am awesome—and here is all the evidence to support that." When do you ever allow yourself to love on yourself this hard? If there were ever a time and a place, it's here and now.

What I accomplished on my Whole30:

30

Today's NSVs

Energy

The Worst   The Best!

1   2   3   4   5   6   7   8   9   10

NOTES: ....

....

Sleep Quality

The Worst   The Best!

1   2   3   4   5   6   7   8   9   10

NOTES: ....

....

Cravings

The Worst   The Best!

1   2   3   4   5   6   7   8   9   10

NOTES: ....

....

FILL IN YOUR OWN

NSV #1: ....

....

....

NSV #2: ....

....

....

NSV #3: ....

....

....

WHAT I ATE

Favorite!

☐ Meal 1: ....

....

....

☐ Meal 2: ....

....

....

☐ Meal 3: ....

....

....

Extra meal/snack: ....

....

....

Day 30 Reflections

....

....

....

....

....

....

....

30

☐ **I did it! Whole30 Day 30 is in the bag.**

REINTRODUCTION 101

Whether you choose the Fast Track or Slow Roll protocol, the three keys to a successful Whole30 reintroduction are: not rushing the process, committing to brutal self-awareness, and taking *really* good notes. We'll give you the basics here, but refer to pages 42–51 and 132–137 in *The Whole30* for detailed guidance.

NOTE: *If this is your first Whole30, we recommend you choose the more structured approach of the Fast Track reintroduction.*

Reintroduction Checklist

Pay attention to all of these areas when you reintroduce off-plan foods, keeping in mind that not all negative effects are physical! If a reintroduced food impacts your motivation or self-confidence, that's worth noting.

- Digestion
- Energy
- Sleep
- Cravings
- Mood and psychology
- Behavior (especially kids)
- Skin
- Breathing
- Pain/inflammation
- Medical conditions/symptoms

TIP

Reintroducing added sugar is tough, because many foods in the other groups will also contain sugar—or enough fast-digesting carbohydrates (like pancakes) to mess with your energy, mood, focus, and cravings. If you want to evaluate sugar all by itself, add a step (and another three days) to your schedule. Keep the rest of your food Whole30-compliant, but add sugar to your morning coffee, drink a full glass of 100% fruit juice mid-morning, top your lunchtime sweet potato with ghee and honey, and pour a generous amount of maple syrup over berries at dinner—then, evaluate energy, mood, focus, hunger, and especially cravings.

FAST TRACK REINTRODUCTION

Summary

The Fast Track Reintroduction schedule is designed to expose you to all previously eliminated food groups in 10 to 14 days, in order of *least likely* to *most likely* be problematic. In our sample schedule, Day 1 is simply the day you decide to move from elimination to reintroduction—it could be your Whole30 Day 31, or a later day if you decided to extend your program. Between each reintroduction day, return to a strict Whole30 diet. Feel free to extend the schedule if you want to break food groups out further (for example, testing corn separately from other non-gluten grains).

Sample Schedule

DAY 1 (OPTIONAL): Evaluate gluten-free alcohol, while keeping the rest of your diet Whole30 compliant. Ex: Red or white wine, 100% agave tequila, gluten-free beer

DAY 1 (OR 4): Evaluate legumes, while keeping the rest of your diet Whole30 compliant. Ex: Peanut butter, edamame or tofu, black beans, hummus

DAY 4 (OR 7): Evaluate non-gluten grains, while keeping the rest of your diet Whole30 compliant. Ex: Gluten-free oats, rice, 100% corn tortillas, gluten-free bread, gluten-free cereal, quinoa

DAY 7 (OR 10): Evaluate dairy, while keeping the rest of your diet Whole30 compliant. Ex: Plain (unsweetened) yogurt, milk or cream, cheese, sour cream

DAY 10 (OR 13): Evaluate gluten-containing grains, while keeping the rest of your diet Whole30 compliant. Ex: Whole wheat cereal, bread, crackers, pasta, beer

My Fast Track Reintroduction

Use this space to plan and record your Fast Track results. While we strongly recommend you follow our order, you are free to reintroduce food groups in the way that works best for you.

DAY 1 Food Group: ....

....

Reintroduced foods: ....

....

....

Days 1–3 Observations: ....

....

....

....

....

....

DAY 4 Food Group: ....

....

Reintroduced foods: ....

....

....

Days 4–6 Observations: ....

....

....

....

....

....

This is called Fast Track, not Shortcut! Don't rush this process, or the negative effects could start to pile up and muddy your evaluation.

DAY 7 Food Group: ....

....

Reintroduced foods: ....

....

....

....

....

Days 7–9 Observations: ....

....

....

....

....

....

....

DAY 10 Food Group: ....

....

Reintroduced foods: ....

....

....

....

....

Days 10–12 Observations: ....

....

....

....

....

....

....

....

DAY 13 Food Group: ....

....

Reintroduced foods: ....

....

....

....

....

Days 13–15 Observations: ....

....

....

....

....

....

....

DAY ____ Food Group: ....

....

Reintroduced foods: ....

....

....

....

....

Days ____ – ____ Observations: ....

....

....

....

....

....

....

DAY ____ Food Group: ⋯⋯⋯⋯⋯⋯⋯⋯⋯⋯⋯⋯⋯⋯⋯⋯⋯⋯⋯
⋯⋯⋯⋯⋯⋯⋯⋯⋯⋯⋯⋯⋯⋯⋯⋯⋯⋯⋯⋯⋯⋯⋯⋯⋯

Reintroduced foods: ⋯⋯⋯⋯⋯⋯⋯⋯⋯⋯⋯⋯⋯⋯⋯⋯⋯
⋯⋯⋯⋯⋯⋯⋯⋯⋯⋯⋯⋯⋯⋯⋯⋯⋯⋯⋯⋯⋯⋯⋯⋯⋯
⋯⋯⋯⋯⋯⋯⋯⋯⋯⋯⋯⋯⋯⋯⋯⋯⋯⋯⋯⋯⋯⋯⋯⋯⋯
⋯⋯⋯⋯⋯⋯⋯⋯⋯⋯⋯⋯⋯⋯⋯⋯⋯⋯⋯⋯⋯⋯⋯⋯⋯
⋯⋯⋯⋯⋯⋯⋯⋯⋯⋯⋯⋯⋯⋯⋯⋯⋯⋯⋯⋯⋯⋯⋯⋯⋯

Days ____ – ____ Observations: ⋯⋯⋯⋯⋯⋯⋯⋯⋯⋯⋯⋯
⋯⋯⋯⋯⋯⋯⋯⋯⋯⋯⋯⋯⋯⋯⋯⋯⋯⋯⋯⋯⋯⋯⋯⋯⋯
⋯⋯⋯⋯⋯⋯⋯⋯⋯⋯⋯⋯⋯⋯⋯⋯⋯⋯⋯⋯⋯⋯⋯⋯⋯
⋯⋯⋯⋯⋯⋯⋯⋯⋯⋯⋯⋯⋯⋯⋯⋯⋯⋯⋯⋯⋯⋯⋯⋯⋯
⋯⋯⋯⋯⋯⋯⋯⋯⋯⋯⋯⋯⋯⋯⋯⋯⋯⋯⋯⋯⋯⋯⋯⋯⋯
⋯⋯⋯⋯⋯⋯⋯⋯⋯⋯⋯⋯⋯⋯⋯⋯⋯⋯⋯⋯⋯⋯⋯⋯⋯

DAY ____ Food Group: ⋯⋯⋯⋯⋯⋯⋯⋯⋯⋯⋯⋯⋯⋯⋯⋯⋯⋯
⋯⋯⋯⋯⋯⋯⋯⋯⋯⋯⋯⋯⋯⋯⋯⋯⋯⋯⋯⋯⋯⋯⋯⋯⋯

Reintroduced foods: ⋯⋯⋯⋯⋯⋯⋯⋯⋯⋯⋯⋯⋯⋯⋯⋯⋯
⋯⋯⋯⋯⋯⋯⋯⋯⋯⋯⋯⋯⋯⋯⋯⋯⋯⋯⋯⋯⋯⋯⋯⋯⋯
⋯⋯⋯⋯⋯⋯⋯⋯⋯⋯⋯⋯⋯⋯⋯⋯⋯⋯⋯⋯⋯⋯⋯⋯⋯
⋯⋯⋯⋯⋯⋯⋯⋯⋯⋯⋯⋯⋯⋯⋯⋯⋯⋯⋯⋯⋯⋯⋯⋯⋯

Days ____ – ____ Observations: ⋯⋯⋯⋯⋯⋯⋯⋯⋯⋯⋯⋯
⋯⋯⋯⋯⋯⋯⋯⋯⋯⋯⋯⋯⋯⋯⋯⋯⋯⋯⋯⋯⋯⋯⋯⋯⋯
⋯⋯⋯⋯⋯⋯⋯⋯⋯⋯⋯⋯⋯⋯⋯⋯⋯⋯⋯⋯⋯⋯⋯⋯⋯
⋯⋯⋯⋯⋯⋯⋯⋯⋯⋯⋯⋯⋯⋯⋯⋯⋯⋯⋯⋯⋯⋯⋯⋯⋯
⋯⋯⋯⋯⋯⋯⋯⋯⋯⋯⋯⋯⋯⋯⋯⋯⋯⋯⋯⋯⋯⋯⋯⋯⋯
⋯⋯⋯⋯⋯⋯⋯⋯⋯⋯⋯⋯⋯⋯⋯⋯⋯⋯⋯⋯⋯⋯⋯⋯⋯

SLOW ROLL REINTRODUCTION

Summary

The Slow Roll Reintroduction schedule doesn't follow any particular timeline. Instead, you'll be eating a mostly Whole30 diet until something so special or delicious-sounding comes along that you decide you're ready to reintroduce that particular food—regardless of the food group it's in. To give you some breathing room, you can relax on the "no added sugar" rule, but *only* with foods unlikely to trigger your sugar dragon. (Ex: deli turkey, meat sticks, chicken sausage, salad dressing, or other condiments.) Here is a sample diary; your days and food choices will vary.

Sample Schedule

DAY 31: Cooking maple bacon with breakfast—nothing else off-plan.

DAY 32: Zero cravings or energy issues from the bacon. Adding this back into regular rotation.

DAY 42: It's my birthday—trying a glass of my favorite red wine with my Whole30 meal, evaluating gluten-free alcohol.

DAY 43: One glass with food had only one negative effect—I *really* wanted a second glass and had to fight that hard.

DAY 47: Movie night—making popcorn with ghee, evaluating corn.

DAY 48: I'm bloated, and the salty crunchy snacks made me crave chocolate! Back to Whole30 until my Sugar Dragon calms down.

DAY 55: Family dinner. Tonight I'm eating mom's homemade pasta.

DAY 56: Digestive distress, headache, tired—back to strict Whole30 for a few days, and gluten is getting a major time-out.

You can continue this indefinitely, slowly adding things that prove worth it (like the maple bacon or one glass of red wine) back to your regular diet until you have a comfortable balance—also known as "food freedom"!

DATE: .... Food group: ....

Food(s) to evaluate: ....
....
....
....
....

Observations: ....
....
....
....
....
....

DATE: .... Food group: ....

Food(s) to evaluate: ....
....
....
....
....

Observations: ....
....
....
....
....

DATE:.. Food group:..

Food(s) to evaluate:...

....

....

....

Observations:...

....

....

....

....

....

DATE:.. Food group:..

Food(s) to evaluate:...

....

....

....

Observations:...

....

....

....

....

....

DATE: .... Food group: ....

....

Food(s) to evaluate: ....

....

....

....

....

Observations: ....

....

....

....

....

....

....

DATE: .... Food group: ....

....

Food(s) to evaluate: ....

....

....

....

....

Observations: ....

....

....

....

....

....

....

....

DATE:.. Food group:..............................

Food(s) to evaluate:...

Observations:...

DATE:.. Food group:..............................

Food(s) to evaluate:...

Observations:...

Melissa's Reflections

Oh hey, Whole30ers . . . YOU DID IT. Thirty days of Whole30, 100% by the book, dramatically changing your health, habits, and relationship with food. It was exciting! It was frustrating. There were easy times and hard times, and days when that seemingly changed by the hour. You laughed, you cursed, you may even have shed a tear over that glorious nacho plate being delivered to the table next to you at your favorite Mexican restaurant. (That was me, actually, during my second Whole30. Literally, I cried. And my table-mate looked at me and said, "Melissa. *It's your own damn program.*")

Later on, as you flip back through this handbook, I hope it serves as a reminder of all the ways you are a strong, capable, confident, healthy person. While some of your reflections may be uncomfortable to revisit, seeing how hard you worked, how far you've come, and how much you've gained throughout the process should fill you with pride.

Let that momentum, strength, and self-confidence carry over into your food freedom. Stay connected to your support system. Follow the Food Freedom plan. Return to this book any time you need a reminder of how capable you truly are. And remember, whenever you need us, the Whole30 community and I will be there to support, encourage, and guide you.

Thank you for sharing your journey with me; I am so proud of what you have done.

Best in health,
Melissa

REFLECTIONS

REFLECTIONS

REFLECTIONS

WHOLE30 RESOURCES

While there are a ton of Whole30 resources available, from cookbooks featuring Whole30 Approved recipes to bloggers who share their Whole30 experience, the only 100% trustworthy sources for Whole30 information come from us—our website, forum, social media feeds, and books. Here's where you can find all the support, motivation, resources, and recipes you'll need to guide your Whole30 journey.

Website

The official home of the Whole30 program. This is where you'll find our free Whole30 Forum, all our free downloads, Whole30 Approved products and affiliates, and more Whole30-related articles than you could possibly hope to read in 30 days. Spend lots of time exploring here before, during, and after your Whole30—this is the very heart of our community.

MAIN SITE: whole30.com

BLOG: whole30.com/blog

FORUM: forum.whole30.com

APPROVED: whole30.com/whole30-approved

RESOURCES: whole30.com/pdf-downloads

Social Media

Our social media channels are incredibly active, featuring the most welcoming, positive community on the entire internet. The Whole30 team, including Melissa, are all very responsive and engaged here too.

FACEBOOK: whole30   TWITTER: @whole30

SNAPCHAT: whole30   ZIING: Whole30

YOUTUBE: whole30   PINTEREST: @whole30

INSTAGRAM: @whole30, @whole30recipes, @whole30approved

Books

It Starts With Food:
Discover the Whole30 and Change Your Life in Unexpected Ways

It Starts With Food shares the "why" behind the Whole30 program, summarizing the science in a simple, accessible manner and revealing how specific foods may be having negative effects on how you look, feel, and live in ways that you'd never associate with your diet. This book introduces our four Good Food standards, explains why the Whole30 eliminates certain food groups, and outlines the health benefits of the foods you are eating on the program.

The Whole30:
The 30-Day Guide to Total Health and Food Freedom

The Whole30 is the complete Whole30 handbook, including planning and preparation tips, an extensive FAQ on meal planning, cravings, troubleshooting, and more, and a huge section on kitchen basics. It also features more than 100 delicious and totally compliant recipes. If you're just looking for the "how," this is where you start.

Food Freedom Forever:
Letting Go of Bad Habits, Guilt, and Anxiety Around Food

Food Freedom Forever offers a detailed plan for creating the perfect diet for you, finding your own healthy balance, and maintaining the kind of control that brings you real food freedom every day. You'll learn how to design your reset, spot your specific triggers before they're pulled, and strategies for dealing with temptation. This book also shares advice for retaining your food freedom during holidays, vacations, periods of life stress, social pressure, and criticism from friends and family.

The Whole30 Cookbook:
150 Delicious and Totally Compliant Recipes to Help You
Succeed with the Whole30 and Beyond

Featuring more than 150 totally compliant recipes (main dishes, sides, dressings, and sauces) to help you prepare delicious, healthy meals during your Whole30 and beyond, The Whole30 Cookbook also offers tips to simplify, plan, and prepare meals to save time and money, and variations to turn one easy dish into two or three meals.

The Whole30 Fast and Easy:
150 Simply Delicious Everyday Recipes for Your Whole30

The Whole30 Fast and Easy makes it even easier to achieve Whole30 success—with delicious, compliant, simple recipes perfect for week-night cooking, lunches in a hurry, and hearty breakfasts that still get you out the door on time. Whether you're doing your first Whole30 or your fifth, or just looking for some healthy, fast, and easy recipes to try, this collection is a must-have for any kitchen.

Meal Planning

Real Plans
w30.co/w30realplans

Delicious, totally compliant Whole30 meals in a weekly plan to fit your taste and schedule. Fully customizable; choose which days of the week and meals to plan, exclude ingredients to which you are allergic or just don't like, and generate an automated shopping list and meal prep instructions for each week. Features 1,000 Whole30-compliant recipes to build into your family's perfect weekly meal plan.

Whole30 Certified Coaches

Work with a Coach
whole30.com/coaches

Our Whole30 Certified Coaching program allows those with the edu-cation, experience, and passion for the Whole30 to lead others through the program in a group (or in some cases, one-on-one) coaching envi-ronment. Our Coaches lead Whole30 group resets, teach seminars, hold cooking and meal prep events, and provide other Whole30 and food freedom services to their local communities. To work with a Coach in your area, visit our website and search by state or zip code.

Whole30 Approved

whole30.com/whole30-approved

This page features a list of our official Whole30 Approved partners. These companies make a variety of products to support your Whole30 journey, and seeing the Whole30 logo on their label means you know you can trust the ingredients and sourcing. However, in many cases, not *every* product they make fits our guidelines. Read your labels, and look for the official Whole30 Approved logo on their website or packaging.

Whole30 Support

Resources to give you Whole30 support, motivation, and accountability.

Wholesome
whole30.com/wholesome

Our free biweekly newsletter filled with Whole30-related advice, tips, recipes, reader stories, discounts, giveaways, and more.

The Whole30 Forum
forum.whole30.com

If you have a question, we can almost guarantee it's been answered. Find those answers, solicit expert advice from our moderators, and get support from fellow Whole30'ers on our free forum.

Whole30 Resources
whole30.com/pdf-downloads

Home to a host of helpful PDF downloads (including our shopping list, meal template, label-reading guide, pantry-stocking guide, and more).

Dear Melissa
whole30.com/category/dear-melissa

My own Whole30 (and life after) advice column, where I answer your questions and share from my own experience.

Connect with Melissa

I love hearing your stories, answering your questions, giving you my best Whole30 and food freedom advice . . . and tough-loving you when you need it.

INSTAGRAM: @melissa_hartwig   FACEBOOK: hartwig.melissa

TWITTER: @melissahartwig_   ZIING: #melissahartwigwhole30